Medical Charting
Demystified

Demystified Series

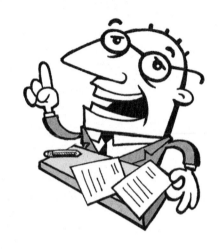

Medical Charting
Demystified

Joan Richards, RN, MSN, CNE
Jim Keogh, RN

New York   Chicago   San Francisco   Lisbon   London
Madrid   Mexico City   Milan   New Delhi   San Juan
Seoul   Singapore   Sydney   Toronto

The McGraw-Hill Companies

1 2 3 4 5 6 7 8 9 0   DOC/DOC   0 1 4 3 2 1 0 9 8

ISBN 978-0-07-149848-7
MHID 0-07-149848-6

Sponsoring Editor
Judy Bass

Proofreader
Medha Joshi

Production Supervisor
Pamela A. Pelton

Indexer
Broccoli Information Management

Editing Supervisor
Stephen M. Smith

Art Director, Cover
Jeff Weeks

Project Manager
Aparna Shukla, International Typesetting
and Composition

Composition
International Typesetting and Composition

Copy Editor
Kathleen McCullough

Printed and bound by RR Donnelley.

McGraw-Hill books are available at special quantity discounts to use as premiums and sales promotions, or for use in corporate training programs. To contact a special sales representative, please visit the Contact Us page at www.mhprofessional.com.

This book is printed on acid-free paper.

This book is dedicated to Eric, whose love, enthusiasm, and spirit inspired me to embark on this meaningful adventure.

—Joan Richards

This book is dedicated to Anne, Sandy, Joanne, Amber-Leigh Christine, and Shawn, without whose help and support this book couldn't have been written.

—Jim Keogh

ABOUT THE AUTHORS

Joan Richards, RN, MSN, CNE, is clinical faculty at New York University College of Nursing, and joint practice clinician at Englewood (N.J.) Hospital and Medical Center.

Jim Keogh, RN, is a member of the faculty at both New York University and Saint Peter's College in New Jersey. He is a registered nurse and is the coauthor of *Medical-Surgical Nursing Demystified, Pharmacology Demystified, Medical Billing and Coding Demystified, Nurse Management Demystified*, and several other books.

CONTENTS AT A GLANCE

CONTENTS

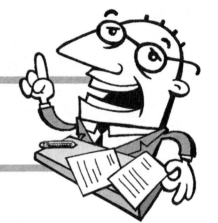

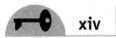

ACKNOWLEDGMENT

We are very thankful to Carol Hefley from McKesson for permitting us to present McKesson's charting software to our readers.

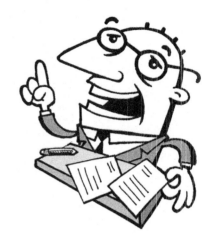

Medical Charting
Demystified

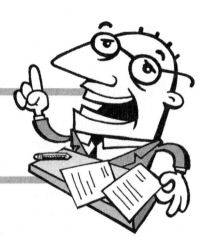

CHAPTER 1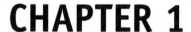

Charting Basics

What's wrong with the patient? What medications has the patient received? Did they work? Questions like these are asked and answered daily by members of the patient's healthcare team as they piece together facts in order to make a diagnosis.

Assessments, test results, and opinions of specialists are some of the facts that lead the healthcare team to determine what's wrong with the patient and the treatments that restore the patient's health. And all are recorded in the patient's chart.

Think of the patient's chart as a database, a body of knowledge about the patient, the one source that has everything the healthcare team needs to return the patient to daily activities of life.

In this chapter, you are introduced to the various styles of charts and learn about the healthcare facilities that use them. You'll also learn what to write in a chart—and what not to write in a chart—and how to avoid common errors and what to do if they should occur.

A Patient's Record

Charting is the task of creating a patient's medical record is called the patient's chart. The chart contains information describing the patient's previous and current medical conditions and healthcare that the patient received and will receive from the healthcare team.

A chart has progressed from a clipboard hanging from the foot of the patient's bed to electronic charts that enable the healthcare team to access and update patient information from computer workstations throughout the healthcare facility and from remote locations. During this transition from paper charts to electronic charts, many healthcare facilities use large loose-leaf binders to hold a patient's record.

The chart is used to document a patient's healthcare and to communicate the patient's medical condition and treatment among the healthcare team. Charting begins when the patient arrives at the healthcare facility when the admitting clerk enters the patient's name, address, medical insurance, and other nonmedical information into the chart.

The nurse completes the admission packet through an interview process. This is where the patient's medical history, social history, current medical problem, current medication list, and the nurse's physical exam, including vital signs, are added to the chart. Next, the physician completes the patient's history and physical and that becomes part of the medical chart. The physician will also write or enter orders for medical tests, treatments, and medications. The healthcare team updates the chart after carrying out each order.

A patient is monitored by a nurse 24 hours a day while in the healthcare facility. Their observations are recorded several times a shift in the patient's chart.

CHARTS BEYOND THE HEALTHCARE TEAM

The patient's chart is used by others besides the healthcare team for purposes other than providing the patient healthcare.

The healthcare facility and the patient's medical insurance carrier use the chart for billing and reimbursements. Medical tests, medications, medical procedures, and other treatments listed in the patient's medical chart are itemized on an invoice prepared by the facility's billing department based on Medicare's Diagnosis-Related Group (DRG). The invoice is submitted to the patient's carrier who refers to the patient's chart to determine if care given to the patient was necessary and customary.

Government agencies and accreditation organizations such as JCAHO (Joint Commission on Accreditation of Healthcare Organizations) audit patients' charts to determine if the healthcare facility and the healthcare team are in compliance with laws and rules designed to assure that patients receive quality healthcare.

Management of the healthcare facility use patients' charts to determine the cost and quality of care and whether or not care is efficiently provided to patients. Charts also serve as a performance baseline and are used by managers and staff to decide if current performance meets acceptable levels.

Medical and nursing students use charts as a puzzle to learn how to care for patients. Students piece together a patient's diagnosis and medical history, physician orders, test results, and progress notes to understand why those orders were issued and how treatment resolved the patient's condition.

Medical researchers find charts contain a treasure trove of raw medical data to study and analyze. They pour over this empirical data looking for clues to improve medical science and patient care.

The patient's chart is key evidence in legal challenges to a patient's medical care. Each element of the chart documents care given to the patient. Attorneys take the position that if care isn't charted, then that care wasn't given to the patient.

Types of Charts

Healthcare institutions adopt a charting system that complements the type of care given to a patient. There are five commonly used charting systems. These are:

Narrative: The narrative charting system begins with the patient health history and assessment. This information is used to develop the patient's care plan that describes details of how the health team will care for the patient. Progress notes (Figure 1-1) and flow sheets are entered in each shift to describe the patient's status and the care that was given to the patient during the shift. The narrative chart concludes with the patient's discharge summary. The narrative charting system is used for ambulatory care, acute care, home care, and long-term care.

Progress Notes
08:30 Patient admitted for complaints of chest pain rated as 8 out of 10 on the pain
scale. Nitroglycerin times 1 administered with relief. Resting quietly at this time.

Figure 1-1

Progress Notes
08:30 S:"I have a lot of pain to a level 10 out of 10" O: Sitting down, grimacing,
clenching fists with movement A: Abdominal pain P: Medicate for pain

Figure 1-2

Problem-Oriented: The problem-oriented charting system focuses on the patient's problems. It too begins with the patient's medical history and assessment. A problem list is created based on the patient's assessment and a care plan is developed that details how the health team is going to address each problem. Progress notes are written at each shift and a discharge summary is prepared for when the patient is discharged. Information is entered into the chart using SOAP, SOAPIE, or SOAPIER formats. SOAP (Figure 1-2) is subjective data (what the patient says), objective data (data based on your observation and testing), assessment data (your conclusion based on subjective and objective data), and plan (your strategy for addressing the patient's problem). SOAPIE (Figure 1-3) is similar except following the plan you record your intervention (the measures that you've taken to care for the patient) and evaluation (the effectiveness of the intervention). The SOAPIER format includes revision (changes to the plan) as the last step. Problem-oriented charting is found in acute, home, and long-term care facilities and in mental health and rehabilitation institution.

Problem-Intervention-Evaluation: Problem-intervention-evaluation charting (Figure 1-4) is focused on ongoing assessment of the patient during each shift. A problem list is created following the patient's history and initial assessment. The patient is then reassessed during each shift and the results are written in progress notes and flow sheets. This charting system is used mainly in acute care facilities.

Progress Notes
08:30 S:"I have a lot of pain to a level 10 out of 10" O: Sitting down, grimacing,
clenching fists with movement A: Abdominal pain P: Medicate for pain I: Medicated
with MS 2 mg IVP E: Patient paint level decreased from 10 to 3 R: Continue with plan

Figure 1-3

Progress Notes
08:30 P: Postoperative nausea I: Medicated with Zofran 4 mg IV E: Nausea subsided:
no further complains.

Figure 1-4

Progress Notes
08:30 D: Questions regarding side effects of new medication A: Explained side effects
of new medication R: Verbalized understanding of potential side effects of new medication

Figure 1-5

FOCUS: FOCUS charting (Figure 1-5) uses a data, action, and response (DAR) format. *Data* refers to what's going on with the patient such as the patient is having difficulty breathing. *Action* is what you did about it such as administration of 2 L of oxygen using a nasal cannula. *Response* is the patient's response to your action such as the patient returned to normal breathing. FOCUS charting requires a patient's history and initial assessment. A checklist of problems (nursing diagnosis) is created and a care plan developed. Flow sheets and progress notes are then used to document patient care. FOCUS charting is frequently seen in acute and long-term care facilities.

Charting by exception is an umbrella term covering the previously mentioned types of charting except for narrative charting, which requires charting of all findings about the patient. The charting by exception style of charting documents abnormal findings using the SOAPIE or SOAPIER format (see Problem-Oriented Charting) or FOCUS charting. The institution establishes standards and norms. Any deviations from these are entered into the chart. Some healthcare facilities find charting by exception efficient and cost effective. The charting by exception chart contains the patient's initial assessment and problem(s). A care plan is developed to address each problem. Flow sheets and progress notes are then used to document the patient's abnormal condition. This charting method is used in acute and long-term care facilities.

COMPONENTS OF A CHART

Each charting system contains a common set of components. These are:

Patient Information: Patient information consists of the patient's name, address, telephone, occupation, employer, insurance carrier, and family contact information.

Patient History: Patient history provides a subjective description of the patient's health and social history. It also contains information about the medical history of the patient's family.

Episodic Information: This component documents the patient's current complaint and initial physical assessment. It answers the question what brought you here today.

Psychosocial Information: Psychosocial information describes the patient's mental and development stage based upon the patient's age. It also describes the patient's current living conditions and social support system, as well as marital status and/or number of children if not a minor.

Medical Orders: The medical orders component contains orders written by healthcare providers. These can be orders for tests, administration of medication, or procedures.

Lab Results: The lab results component identifies the laboratory tests that were performed and the results of those tests.

Tests Results: There can be one or more sections of the chart for test results depending on the charting system adopted by the healthcare facility. Some charting systems will have a section for commonly performed tests such as electrocardiogram (ECG), or diagnostics for x-rays Test results usually contain the numeric or graphical results and a narrative that describes the examiner's findings.

Progress Notes: A progress note describes an observation made by a healthcare provider, such as a physician, relating to the patient's care.

Nurses' Notes: Nurses' notes contain observations of the patient made by the patient's primary nurse. Many hospitals now utilize the multidisciplinary progress note so that all providers from the healthcare team are charting on the same record and the information is shared.

Care Plan: The care plan describes details on how the healthcare team will address the patient's problems.

Legal: The legal component of the chart contains patient consent forms, living will, advanced directives, and other legal documents that direct how the patient wants to be cared for while in the healthcare facility.

Medication Administration Report (MAR): The MAR contains the record of medication ordered for the patient and when it was administered. Information on the MAR is pulled from the medical orders component of the chart.

Discharge Information: The discharge information component contains a checklist of things to do when discharging the patient and a record of whether or not it was performed. It also contains instructions that the nurse must give the patient before the patient leaves the healthcare facilities.

TIP *An incident report is NOT part of the patient's chart. An incident report must be written for errors and potential errors that occur during the patient's care (see Chapter 2).*

Writing in a Chart

It is important to keep in mind that you are telling the patient's story when you write a chart. You're telling members of the healthcare team and others who are involved with the patient information about the patient's health and the care that the healthcare team delivered to the patient.

The nursing process, referred to as ADPIE, is a good approach to follow when documenting patient care. ADPIE is the acronym for assessment, diagnose, plan, intervention, and evaluation.

Assessment is the systematic collection of data and verifying the collected data. That is, symptoms reported by the patient are independently verified through observations and testing.

A *diagnosis* is the identification of the patient's problem by looking for data clusters that lead to a pattern pointing to a problem. There are two kinds of diagnoses: medical and nursing. This difference becomes evident when using the ADPIE type of charting, which focuses only on the nursing diagnosis.

The *plan* details how the healthcare team will treat the patient. It lists who will do what and when it will be done. The plan is described in medical orders and in the patient's care plan and serves as a map guiding the healthcare team as they resolve the patient's healthcare problem.

Intervention is carrying out the plan. Each step of the plan that is performed is documented in the chart. The time, date, route, and who administered medications are entered into the MAR (see Medication Administration Report). Test results are entered into the chart along with interpretation of those results depending on the test. All interventions must be documented in the chart. The absence of documentation means that the intervention was not performed.

Evaluation describes what happened after the intervention. Did the intervention resolve the patient's problem? The evaluations of interventions are documented in progress notes, nurse's notes, and flow sheets. The healthcare team may continue, modify, or terminate the plan for treating the patient depending on the evaluation.

RULES FOR CHARTING

The patient's life depends greatly on how well the patient's chart is written. What may be simple, understandable errors such as illegible and slightly misspelled words can have a grave effect on a patient's care.

Everything written in a chart must be legible. This is crucial if charting is not performed using a computer and instead entries are written. Countless errors occur when healthcare providers scribble orders, test results, or progress notes in order to quickly move on to the next patient.

Don't assume. Illegible charting leaves others on the healthcare team one of two choices: guess at the meaning of what was written or verify it by contacting the healthcare team member who wrote it. Unfortunately, an educated guess often overrides the time-consuming task of trying to verify the order, which can lead to fatal errors.

Does it make sense? Take a moment and stop a second. Ask yourself if what you intend to document makes sense in terms of the patient's health. Is what you are about to write is clearly related to the patient's problem, treatment plan, or intervention? The chart should only contain concise relative information.

Only accurate facts should be entered into the chart. Chart your opinion, only state the facts as they present themselves. Others on the healthcare team are basing their decisions on what you write in the chart. It is always better to write facts that you personally observed. Always provide facts that lead you to any conclusion.

Chart in a timely fashion. Ideally chart at the bedside. If this is not possible, then chart immediately after you leave the patient when the information is fresh in your mind. Any delay in charting can lead to errors. You may not recall the information about your patient or you might confuse the information with information about another patient. Others on the healthcare team may make decisions about the patient based on outdated information.

Watch your spelling! Changing one letter in a word can have an altogether different meaning and have serious repercussions for the patient. Don't guess at a spelling or phonetically spell a word. Take the time to look up the correct spelling.

Avoid abbreviations. Abbreviations save time and space when charting; however, abbreviations are the source of errors because the assumption is that everyone who reads a chart knows the meanings of abbreviations. It is always best to avoid using abbreviations when charting. Healthcare facilities always have a list of approved abbreviations for that institution.

Chart only for yourself. Don't chart for other members of the healthcare team because you did not observe those facts yourself.

Date and sign each entry. Begin each entry into the chart with the time and date. Document your findings and then sign the entry followed by your title.

Be complete in your charting. Specify an intervention and evaluation for each problem that you document. If you write that the patient has difficulty breathing, then be sure to write what you did to solve the problem.

TIP *It is best to use black ink when charting. Black ink shows up better when charts are photocopied or faxed.*

VERBAL ORDERS

Physicians and other members of the healthcare team who are authorized to issue orders must explicitly write those orders in the patient's chart. In extreme emergencies, a nurse can take verbal orders over the telephone, which is then followed up with written orders once the healthcare provider arrives at the healthcare facility.

Here are guidelines to follow when taking verbal orders.

Don't accept a verbal order if the healthcare provider is in the healthcare facility unless there is a system in place that directs the physician to enter the order into the computer or write the order in the chart within 24 hours of giving the verbal order. Always know the correct policy for your institution for guidelines related to taking verbal orders.

Ask the healthcare provider to fax the order if possible. The fax should contain the healthcare provider's signature. Always know the correct policy for your institution for guidelines related to faxing printed orders.

Read back the order to the physician to avoid errors when taking verbal orders.

Write down the order during the call. Make sure the patient is correctly identified and the right medication, dose, routine, and time are indicated if it is an order for medication.

Clarify any portion of the order that doesn't make sense. Ask the healthcare provider to spell the patient's name and names of medications. Realize that the healthcare provider can be mistaken.

Verify the order by reading what you wrote to the healthcare provider. Also compare the verbal order to information in the patient's chart to assure you are dealing with the correct patient and that the order doesn't conflict with current orders.

Talk directly to the healthcare provider. Don't take verbal orders from anyone who is not authorized to issue an order.

Write the verbal order in the chart. Sign the healthcare provider's name followed by your name indicating that this is a verbal order. The healthcare provider must countersign the order within 24 hours.

What to Write

Your objective is to clearly report on the patient's progress using as few words as possible. That is, make your point and avoid writing everything that went on in the patient's life that day. Your writing provides other members of the healthcare team facts about the patient that helps them continue caring for the patient.

It is critical to chart facts and not your opinion. For example, "had a good day" or "did not appear to be in that much pain" are opinions, not facts. On the other hand, "patient reported a pain of 2 (0–10)" is fact.

Likewise, charting "physician was called" is a fact; however, "when I called the physician about this patient, he sounded tired and not interested in what I had to say" is an opinion.

Avoid writing words that could defame someone. Charting is not the place to attack the good name and reputation of the patient or anyone on the healthcare team.

Throughout this book we'll show techniques of keeping your charting to the minimum amount of words while still conveying important facts about the patient. It isn't easy to keep your notes brief and to the point. For example, Figure 1-6 shows a rather long-winded way to chart the patient's pain. A better description is shown in Figure 1-7.

A common trick used by experienced nurses is to draw a mental picture of the patient's problem and then describe that image in the chart. Let's say that you are describing a wound. Picture the wound in your mind and then describe the wound in the chart such as "large abdominal dressing intact with 1 cm of red/brown wound drainage noted."

Another trick is to think logically and systematically when charting. Use a head to toe approach and describe each system completely before moving on to the next system. This is illustrated in Figure 1-8 where the progress notes begin with the neurological system and then to the respiratory system.

Progress Notes
08:30 patient complained about a lot of pain and when I asked what the number
was on the pain scale, he said that it was a 10.

Figure 1-6

Progress Notes
08:30 Complaints of pain; 10 on 1–10 pain scale

Figure 1-7

Progress Notes
08:30 sleepy but responsive to name and vigorous stimulation; pupils sluggish but
reative to light. Anterior lungs clear to auscultation with rhonchi heard across
lung fields; clears with coughing.

Figure 1-8

Fixing Errors

Expect to make errors when writing in a chart because it happens to everyone. Typically, you are adding information on a page that already contains information entered by others on the healthcare team; therefore simply ripping up the page and starting over isn't an option when you entered an error on the chart.

Instead you must draw a single line through the error and place your initials above the line. Don't cover up the error with white out or heavily cross out the text making it unreadable. The error must be legible and clearly indicate it is an error. Making the error illegible might lead someone to believe that the error is being concealed.

TIP *Visitors and relatives are not authorized to see the chart. Never leave the chart open or visible to unauthorized personnel (see HIPAA in Chapter 2).*

Summary

Charting is the task of creating a patient's medical record called the patient's chart. The chart contains information describing the patient's previous and current medical conditions and healthcare that the patient received and will receive from the healthcare team.

Charts are used for purposes other than providing patient healthcare. They are used for billing, reimbursements by medical insurance carriers, accreditation and licensed organizations, managing the healthcare facility, legal matters, and researching and learning about patient care.

There are two commonly used charting systems. Charting systems are either narrative or problem-focused charting by exception which is now most commonly used. When using the charting by exception method, the nurse can choose between one of three common types of problem charting which are problem-oriented, problem-intervention-evaluation, and FOCUS. The institution where you work will have a policy that indicates the type of charting used in that institution for nursing and other healthcare providers. Each of these systems has common components that provide general information about the patient including the patient's medical history, current problem, assessments, test results, diagnosis, medical orders, treatment plan, and discharge teachings.

When writing in a chart it is important that you keep in mind that you are telling the patient's story to other members of the healthcare team. Write legibly. Present only facts. Make sure what you write makes sense. If you make an error, draw a single line through the error and initial it.

Quiz

1. At change of shift, the nurse you are relieving forgot to update the patient's chart with the latest vitals. She gives you a slip of paper and asks you to enter it into the chart. What is the best response?

   a. Enter the vitals as requested.

   b. Say that you'll do it this time only.

   c. Take your own set of vitals and enter it into the chart.

   d. Explain that policy requires each nurse to do their own charting.

2. You are supervising a student nurse who makes an error when charting progress notes. What should you do?

   a. Explain that errors occur and the draw a single line through the error and initial it.

   b. Explain that errors occur and give the nursing student a new page to rewrite everything that is on the page that contains the error.

   c. Explain that errors are not acceptable and order the student nurse off the floor.

   d   Explain that the error information is close to being correct and it won't matter because the patient is being discharged anyway.

3. You are reviewing a patient's chart and notice a component that doesn't belong in the chart. Which of the following should be removed from the chart?

   a. Care plan

   b. Medical insurance information

c.   Opinions from a specialist who reviews test results

   d.   An incident report

4. A nurse is called to testify in a malpractice case. The patient's attorney claims the chart shows that the important treatment was ordered but nothing in the chart shows that it was performed by the nurse. The hospital's attorney places the nurse on the stand to testify that she performed the treatment. What is the judge likely conclude?

   a.   The treatment was performed but not charted.

   b.   The nurse is lying.

   c.   The treatment wasn't performed because it wasn't charted.

   d.   Charting the treatment is irrelevant to the case.

5. A new nurse asks what abbreviations can be used in a chart. The best response is.

   a.   Review hospital policy.

   b.   Only use abbreviations that are found in standard nursing textbooks.

   c.   Never use any abbreviations.

   d.   Always use abbreviations to save time and space in the chart.

6. A new nurse is having difficulty reading a medical order in the patient's chart. What is the best course of action to take?

   a.   Ask another nurse to help interpret the written order.

   b.   Ask another nurse supervisor to help interpret the written order.

   c.   Call the healthcare provider who wrote the order for clarification.

   d.   Ask the physician on call to interpret the written order.

7. After administering scheduled medication, where would you document it in the chart?

   a.   Medication administration report

   b.   Progress notes

   c.   Nurse's notes

   d.   Update the care plan

8. Which of the following isn't appropriate to write in a chart?

   a.   The patient had a bad day and won't get out of bed to exercise.

   b.   The patient in bed, two rails up.

   c.   The patient refused to eat breakfast, saying that he wasn't hungry.

   d.   135/70, R 20, P 72, T 98.7

9. A student nurse asks how the patient's chart is used for reimbursement of medical expenses. The best response is

   a. The patient's diagnosis is listed in the chart and is compared to Medicare's Diagnosis-Related Group, which is used to determine reimbursements of medical expenses.

   b. The billing department faxes the entire chart to the medical insurance company for review.

   c. The billing department reviews the chart to itemize all the expenses related to caring for the patient.

   d. The chart is not used for reimbursement of medical expenses.

10. A student nurse asks how a patient's chart can be used to learn about patient care. The best response is

   a. You can piece together assessments and test results to see how the healthcare provider diagnosed the patient and then see why specific medications and treatments were prescribed to address the patient's problem.

   b. You can look up medical words and tests you see in the chart, so you understand what is happening to the patient.

   c. After reviewing the chart, you can call the healthcare provider and ask why medications and treatments that are listed in the chart were prescribed.

   d. The chart isn't a good tool to use to learn about patient care.

CHAPTER 2

The Legal Aspect of Charting

The difference between a successful malpractice law suit and the case being dismissed can be the contents of the patient's chart. Judges and jurors who must determine facts in a malpractice action weigh the patient's chart heavily in their decisions because it is a record of what did occur and what didn't occur in the care of the patient.

A properly worded and carefully written chart that conforms to healthcare standards implies that the healthcare team went to great pains to provide the patient with a level of care that everyone can expect to receive.

An inappropriately documented chart that fails to adhere to standards shouts to everyone that the patient might have received substandard care from the healthcare team and they therefore might be guilty of malpractice or other violations of the patient's rights.

In this chapter, you'll learn what is appropriate and inappropriate charting. You'll also learn how to avoid common charting mistakes that give a defense attorney reason to believe that the healthcare team mishandled caring for the patient.

A Patient's Record and the Law

The patient's chart is a confidential record of the patient's condition and treatment and is protected by ethical and legal regulations that define how and by whom it can be used. The goal of these regulations is to give patients control of their healthcare information and to limit access to patient information to those who provide care to the patient. This includes physicians, nurses, medical insurers, and administrators who are involved in billing, reimbursement, and managing the healthcare facility.

LIMITED ACCESS

The patient's chart contains a wealth of information about the patient. It is a database of the patient's health history; personal information such as name, address, identification numbers, and the patient's diagnosis; treatment; tests results; and care that healthcare providers plan to deliver to the patient.

Each person who is involved with the patient's care is permitted to access just the patient's data that is necessary to deliver their service rather than access to the complete chart. For example, a pharmacist needs information about the patient to provide proper medication, but doesn't need to know the patient's address or billing information. Patient confidentiality extends to discussing information about the patient to others who are not directly involved in the patient's care, including casual conversations with colleagues.

Information about a patient can be shared with colleagues as long as the patient's identity remains confidential. Nurses can ask a colleague for suggestions on how to intervene in a specific condition that affects a patient without revealing the identity of the patient.

TIP *Patients have the right to see their charts and other parts of their medical records. The healthcare facility has a policy that describes the procedures for releasing this information to patients.*

UNKNOWINGLY VIOLATING CONFIDENTIALITY

However, concealing the patient's identity isn't as simple as not mentioning the patient's name or room number. Patient confidentiality is violated if the colleague can piece together information given by the nurse.

Suppose the nurse asks a colleague about interventions for a patient with prostrate problems. If there is only one male patient in the unit 50 years old or older, then it is easy to determine the patient to whom the nurse refers.

Other clues to the patient's identity are age, gender, diagnosis, physician (if the physician has only one patient on the unit), usual event (i.e., one patient on the unit acted out), nationality, race, and handicap.

PROTECTING THE PATIENT

Nurses are obligated to guard against unauthorized access to the patient's chart while the patient is in the unit. The nurse must immediately challenge anyone who requests a chart or who is seen reviewing the chart if that person is not involved with the patient's care.

It is also critical that the patient's identity is protected from public display. This becomes a balancing act between the need to protect patient confidentiality and the need for members of the healthcare team to identify the patient.

For example, some healthcare facilities post staff patient assignments on a large white board near the nurse's station or at the entrance to the unit. This enables the staff to quickly identify who is responsible for a patient's care. Only the nurse's first name, the patient's initials, and the room number maybe listed. More details might be available on a clipboard at the nurse's station.

Hint: Always place a blank sheet of paper as the top sheet of the clipboard.

The challenge is to identify the patient without violating patient confidentiality. Using room and bed numbers to identify a patient is a JCAHO (Joint Commission on Accreditation of Healthcare Orgainzations) violation. Some facilities use the patient's first name and initial of the last name.

A similar problem exists with identifying charts if the facility isn't using computerized charting; even with computerized charting, there is always a paper chart. Paper charts are usually stored in a large loose-leaf binder at the nurse's station or in a mobile cart used during rounds. The patient's identity must appear on the spine of the loose-leaf binder. Facilities commonly label the chart with the room and bed number.

Tip *Can the patient see his or her chart? Yes. Patients can receive a copy of their medical records and the patient can ask for amendments. The healthcare facility typically has a policy that describes the procedure for the patient to review the chart.*

HIPAA

The Health Insurance Portability and Accountability Act (HIPAA) is the primary legislation that governs the use of a patient's medical record. HIPAA establishes rules for securing and managing a patient's healthcare records as well as coding and reimbursements.

Healthcare providers are required to inform their patients about HIPAA's privacy requirements and ask patients to sign an acknowledgement that they were notified by the healthcare provider. Patients also must be asked to sign a consent allowing the healthcare provider to share the patients' medical records for routine medical care.

In keeping with the goal of patient confidentiality, HIPAA requires that patient information be disclosed on a need-to-know basis. The healthcare provider must explain to patients how they maintain the required patient confidentiality.

TIP *The patient has the right to restrict the kind of information that is shared and with whom it is shared.*

Charting to Limit Legal Liability

The patient's chart is the cornerstone to many malpractice actions because it describes the patient's condition, diagnosis, and care while the patient was in the healthcare facility. Inaccurate or incomplete documentation indicates to a judge and jury that the patient received below standard care by the healthcare team. Therefore, the best defense against a malpractice suit is a good offense by accurately documenting patient care.

The objective is to chart exactly the patient's assessment and treatment immediately and in terms that leave no doubt in the reader's mind as to what occurred. Describe the patient's problem (assessment), what you did to address the problem (intervention), and how the patient reacted (outcome). Excluding any of these leaves the chart incomplete and opened to speculation by attorneys, judges, and jurors.

TIP *If it isn't charted, then it didn't happen.*

TARGETS OF MALPRACTICE ATTORNEYS

The purpose of charting is not to avoid a law suit, but to provide factual information about the patient to members of the healthcare team. In doing so, you'll provide consistent and comprehensive information, which is also the best way to defend a malpractice case.

Standards for charting are defined by a number of organizations and laws. These are the Nurse Practice Acts, which define the scope of practice for nurses; the American Nurses Association (ANA), whose standards are used to accredit the healthcare facility; and the facility's own policy.

Experienced attorneys focus on common errors that occur in charting and then exploit them as proof that malpractice has occurred. You can reduce exposure to legal action by making sure that you avoid these errors.

Here's what you need to do:

Correct errors in the chart immediately, otherwise the error can lead to additional errors.

Don't make errors in the chart illegible. The assumption will be that you are hiding something. Draw a single line through the error and initial it using the same black pen that was used to write the incorrect information in the chart. This shows that you recognized your error and corrected it immediately.

Don't chart in advance. Although doing so saves time, it is also risky because you may be distracted and not provide the treatment.

Don't enter the incorrect time. Patient load sometimes prevents you from providing treatment when it is scheduled. This can have serious ramifications, especially when administering medication.

Don't write critical comments or opinions in the chart. Simply write the objective facts using acceptable medical terminology and let the reader draw a conclusion based on those facts.

Don't leave any blank space between what you write and your signature. This leaves the opportunity for someone else to add information to what you've charted. Draw a line through the space if you can't avoid leaving a space.

Enter verbal orders in the chart immediately and make sure that the physician signs them. Verbal orders that don't appear in the chart are considered not ordered.

Don't skip lines when charting. All your information must be on consecutive lines.

Always use black ink. Attempts to alter the chart will easily be noticed.

Don't allude in the chart to the filing of an incident report.

Make sure that you perform a complete assessment of the patient and chart your results. Failure to do so can be construed as breach of duty.

Avoid mentioning other patients in the chart because this violates patient confidentiality.

Always document the patient's response and comments by placing the patient's exact words in quotations.

Make sure you are entering accurate information into the correct patient's chart. It is best to take a 10-second time out to give yourself a moment to collect yourself before writing anything in the chart.

Don't carry out orders that you question. Document that you called the physician for clarification for the specific order. Be sure to note the date and time.

Always chart instructions given to the patient when the patient is discharged and chart whether or not the patient understood those discharge instructions (Figure 2-1). Also, chart if the patient was not able to demonstrate or verbalize the discharge instruction; however, you'll need to chart your intervention, such as re-educate the patient.

Avoid using words that imply that an error occurred.

TIP Chart anything that might be important in malpractice litigation.

Progress Notes
08:30 patient verbalized understanding of discharge instruction related to wound care

Figure 2-1

Elements of Malpractice

The patient's chart is a key element that determines if a patient's malpractice action is successful. The court and jurors examine the chart to determine if the patient received the standard care from the healthcare team. The standard of care is defined by a number of legal and accreditation organizations. However, the standard tested in the courts is whether or not a reasonable and equally trained member of the healthcare team having similar experience would have acted the same as the defendant in caring for the patient.

The patient's attorney sets out to prove that the patient was injured (damage) because of the medical team's action (causation) or inaction (breach of duty), which demonstrates negligence when caring for the patient. That is, the healthcare team did something that should not have been performed or didn't do something that should have been performed according to standard care. Malpractice is a form of negligence that stipulates that a professional did not act reasonably and in good faith while performing a service to another person. In other words, a member of the healthcare team did not respond the way another professional may have responded.

Say that a patient received a urinary tract infection from catherization. A member of the healthcare team injured the patient. Whether or not this was malpractice or not depends on a number of factors.

Did the patient consent to the procedure?

Was the patient informed of the risks of performing the procedure?

Did the physician order the procedure?

Was the nurse who performed the procedure trained, validated, licensed, and authorized by the healthcare facility to perform the procedure?

Did the nurse have reason to believe that the equipment was sterile and working properly?

Did the nurse adhere to the standards when performing the procedure?

If the answers are yes, then malpractice didn't occur. However, answering no to any of these questions raises the question of malpractice because there is a failure to meet the standard of care that the patient is entitled to receive.

Attorneys compare the patient's chart, the facility's policies, the healthcare team's background, and standards established by legal and accrediting organizations to the treatment that the patient received to prove their case of malpractice.

TIP *Communicate often with the patient during treatment to maintain the nurse-patient relationship so you can address any perceived dissatisfaction with care before the patient seeks legal remedies.*

Writing an Incident Report

An incident report documents a serious exception to normal procedures. These exceptions may be dangerous or may lead to potential litigation. The policies of the healthcare facility describe situations when an incident report must be filed with the Risk Management Department or the appropriate department within the facility. Never place an incident report in the patient's chart; however, the incident report can be used as evidence in litigation.

The Risk Management Department then conducts its own investigation and reports the results to the healthcare facility's attorney and insurance carrier. The situation leading up to and the handling of the incident are reviewed by management in order to improve procedures depending on the nature of the incident.

Each person who is involved in the incident, including those who witnessed all or part of the incident, should file an incident report that describes the facts of the incident according to their first-hand observations.

In writing the incident report, you should:

Write your own incident report on forms provided by the healthcare facility. Use additional pages if needed.

Make sure to identify the patient, the time and place of the incident, and what you did once you became aware of the incident.

Describe how the incident affected the patient.

Don't leave blank spaces on the incident report. Draw a single line through any blank spaces. This prevents anyone from inserting facts to the incident report that you didn't write.

Don't write your observations on someone else's incident report.

Write only facts that you identified. If you didn't see it, then don't write about it—no assumptions or opinions. Let others draw a conclusion from the facts.

Make sure facts in the chart coincide with facts in the incident report.

Specify what you did when you encountered the incident.

Write in quotations whatever the patient or others say to you.

Don't blame anyone for the incident. Let the facts speak for themselves.

Other Legal Documents
Part of the Patient's Chart

The patient's chart contains legal documents that authorize or acknowledge the patient's wishes regarding treatment. These are informed consent, advance directives, and a refusal of treatment. The informed consent authorizes the medical team to perform a specific procedure or administer a specific treatment to the patient. An advance directive tells the healthcare team the patient's wishes for care should the patient become incapacitated and unable to communicate. Refusal of treatment acknowledges that the patient is rejecting prescribed medical care.

Each of these documents must be signed by the patient; however, before doing so the healthcare provider must explain to the patient the benefits and risks of the prescribed course of action and alternative options including not doing anything.

The patient must be legally competent and have the capability to fully comprehend what is being asked of him or her. The test of this is to have the patient repeat in the patient's own words what the healthcare provider explained.

Once the healthcare provider is confident that the patient understands, then the patient is asked to sign the document and the healthcare provider countersigns it as a witness to the patient's signature.

Only patients who are legally competent can sign the document, otherwise a guardian such as a parent or court-appointed representative can sign on behalf of the patient. Healthcare facilities have clear policies on who can sign these documents.

INFORMED CONSENT

An informed consent authorizes the healthcare team to perform procedures on the patient. It is the physician's responsibility to have the patient sign the informed consent. Before the patient signs the consent form, the physician must provide the patient with information necessary for the patient to make an informed decision to either undergo the prescribed treatment or opt for alternative treatment or no treatment at all.

It is common for the nurse, in the role as a patient advocate, to make sure that a consent form has been signed by the patient. The nurse asks the patient if the patient understood the healthcare provider's explanation about the diagnoses, prescribed treatment, and the risks involved in the treatment. In addition, the nurse asks if the healthcare provider discussed alternative treatments and the risk for each.

Encourage the patient to ask questions and then answer them or have the healthcare provider return to further explain the proposed procedure. It is the healthcare provider's responsibility to explain the treatment to the patient and obtain the patient's consent. It is not the nurse's responsibility. The nurse is responsible for making sure that the patient understands the procedure. The nurse might be asked to witness the patient signing the consent form. If this happens, the nurse also signs the consent form as a witness.

It is critical that the patient also understands that the consent is only for a particular treatment. Current treatment continues even if the patient doesn't sign the consent form and that he will still be offered future treatment regardless if the consent form is signed.

Additionally, the patient must be told that consent can be withdrawn at anytime even after the consent form is signed. The patient can simply tell the healthcare provider to stop and treatment will be stopped.

Patients must sign the consent form of their own free will based on all the options presented to them by the healthcare provider. Failure to objectively present the benefits and risks of all the treatment alternatives can be construed as coercion and might nullify the signed consent form. The healthcare team might be committing a battery if treatment is given without a valid signed consent form.

Once the consent form is signed and countersigned as witness to the signature, the consent form is placed in the patient's chart. Document in the nurse's notes that the patient confirmed the healthcare provider gave the patient information about treatments and options prior to signing the consent form.

Also, document that the patient refused to sign the consent form. Explicitly describe your actions and the patient's response. Make sure that you document the patient's actual words using quotations and document what you did after the patient refused to sign, such as contacting the nurse manager and the healthcare provider, and steps taken to prevent the treatment from beginning.

The patient must consent before any procedure is performed, including routine procedures that are covered by the general consent form signed when the patient is admitted to the healthcare facility. Consent for routine procedures such as inserting a urinary catheter can be given orally. However, the patient must still be told of why the healthcare providers wants the procedure performed, the benefits and risks associated with it, and options to performing the procedure.

There are two situations when a signed informed consent is not necessary. These are in an emergency and if the patient isn't interested in hearing about the treatment.

TIP *If the patient can't explain the proposed treatment to you, then stop. Further explanation is needed from the healthcare provider.*

ADVANCE DIRECTIVES

An advance directive is a legal document signed by the patient that gives the healthcare team instructions about how the patient wants life-sustaining care should the patient be unable to convey his or her wishes.

Patients can request not to be resuscitated if the patient experiences cardiac arrest or respiratory arrest or to be disconnected from life-supporting equipment if there is no hope for the patient's survival.

The patient can change the advance directive at any time by telling the healthcare provider that he or she no longer wants the advance directive enforced. The healthcare facility will have a policy describing how to document the patient request to change the advance directive.

Any legally competent adult can create an advance directive. It must be signed and the signature witnessed. Terms of the advance directive must comply with legal restrictions, which may define basic care (i.e., nutrients) that must be given to all patients regardless of their wishes.

Some patients already have an advance directive prior to being admitted to the healthcare facility. If so, then a copy of it must be placed in the patient's chart and so documented in the nurse's notes.

Upon admission, the patient is always asked if they have an advance directive. If they do not have one, information about initiating a directive is given to the patient. After reading the information, the patient can either ask for a directive to complete or continue to refuse the option. The nurse will indicate on the admission charting, the patient's response to the directive offer. You might be required to witness the patient's signature. If so, then document the patient's mental state in the nurse's notes. This becomes evidence that the patient was competent at the time the advance directive was created.

Failure to comply with terms of an advance directive can expose the healthcare team to legal action by the patient or the patient's family.

TIP The advance directive is followed only when the patient is unable to speak for himself or herself.

There are two types of advance directives. These are living wills and durable power of attorney.

A living will specifies the kind of care the patient wants to receive if he or she becomes incapacitated requiring extraordinary measures (i.e., feeding tube, ventilator) to sustain the patient's life.

A durable power of attorney designates a person to make healthcare decisions for the patient if the patient becomes unable to make decisions for himself or herself.

TIP Make sure that you know how to contact the designated person. Contact information in the durable power of attorney may be outdated unless it was recently created.

It is important for the physician to review the patient's advance directive if the patient is at risk for becoming comatose or arresting. The physician will write a

DNR order if the physician feels that the patient understands the impact of the DNR order. However, the physician may choose not to write the DNR order. If this happens, you need to document this in the nurse's notes.

TIP *Don't call a code if the patient has a DNR order.*

Some healthcare facilities clearly mark DNR on the spine of the patient's chart that has a do not resuscitate provision in the patient's advance directive so that the healthcare team can respond appropriately in an emergency.

The DNR order should be reviewed with the patient frequently and especially when the patient's condition changes, especially for the better. The patient may want to rescind the DNR request. Healthcare facilities have policies that specify how to handle a DNR order.

Typically, DNR orders must be reviewed and renewed by the physician every 72 hours. Don't accept a verbal DNR order. Every DNR order must be written.

TIP *Always let the nurse manager, physician, the healthcare facility's legal department, or other appropriate department handle advance directives issues.*

Many hospitals have variations of the DNR order; for instance, the do not intubate (DNI) order. This is a DNR order that enables the physician to take lifesaving measures up until the point of intubation. There is no in between.

REFUSAL OF TREATMENT

A legally competent patient has the right to refuse treatment and can request to be discharged against medical advice (AMA). Healthcare facilities typically have a Refuse Treatment form and a Discharge Against Medical Advice form, which the patient is requested to sign releasing the healthcare team from liability.

The patient can refuse complete treatment or an aspect of the treatment such as insertion of a urinary catheter. When this occurs, the physician is required to explain to the patient the benefits of the treatment and the risk of not undergoing treatment. Once the physician is convinced the patient is making an informed decision, then the patient is presented with the Refuse Treatment form.

The Refuse Treatment form describes the patient's diagnosis and treatment and acknowledges that the physician explained the risk of failing to undergo treatment. The patient is asked to sign the form, which is countersigned by a witness. The form is then placed in the patient's chart.

A similar process occurs when the patient is discharged against medical advice. The Discharge Against Medical Advice form must contain the patient's own words stating that he wants to leave and the risk of leaving. Furthermore, the form must also identify the physician who explained the risk to the patient.

Although the patient is free to leave the healthcare facility, the healthcare team is required to provide support to the patient by giving the patient written directions for follow-up medical care, such as at the clinic, and notify the patient's family that the patient is leaving against medical advice and might require additional support at home.

It is important to document recommended follow-up support, which relatives were notified, where the patient is going after being discharged, and who accompanied the patient leaving the healthcare facility.

Document in the nurse's notes whenever a patient refuses treatment or is discharged against medical advice. Be sure to record the patient's mental state and exact words and what you did after the patient made the request.

There might be occasions when the patient refuses to sign these forms. You can't force the patient to sign any form. Healthcare facilities have policies on how to respond to such situations. Typically, the physician and another member of the healthcare team will witness the patient's refusal and then note that in the patient's chart (nurse's notes or progress notes). Some healthcare facilities ask that a member of the patient's family to sign the form as confirmation of the patient's intent.

TIP Ask the physician to explain to the patient each aspect of the planned treatment immediately after the patient is admitted. This gives the physician time to provide alternatives to the treatment plan should the patient refuse all or part of the treatment.

WHERE'S THE PATIENT?

There is bound to be a time when the patient simply leaves the healthcare facility without telling anyone. This is called patient elopement. Most healthcare facilities have a policy that lists steps to take once the patient is noticed missing. Typically, you'll contact security and your supervisor before calling the patient's family and the police.

It is important for you to document this entire event objectively and in chronological order. Describe when and how you discovered the patient missing and how you responded—who and when you called for assistance (i.e., security, supervisor, and police) and their response. Record the event so that anyone reading it is able to retrace your steps.

Summary

The patient's chart is a confidential record of the patient's condition and treatment and is protected by ethical and legal regulations that define how it can be used and by whom. The goal is to give patients control of their healthcare information and to limit access to patient information to those who provide care to the patient.

Each person who is involved with the patient's care is permitted to access just the patient's data that are necessary to deliver their service rather than access to the complete chart. Nurses are obligated to guard against unauthorized access to the patient's chart while the patient is in the unit. The Health Insurance Portability and Accountability Act (HIPAA) is the primary legislation that governs the use of a patient's medical record.

The purpose of charting is not to avoid a law suit, but to provide factual information about the patient to members of the healthcare team. The court and jurors examine the chart to determine if the patient received the standard of care from the healthcare team.

An incident report documents a serious exception to normal procedures. An advance directive tells the healthcare team the patient's wishes for care should the patient become incapacitated and unable to communicate. An informed consent authorizes the healthcare team to treat the patient. A legally competent patient has the right to refuse treatment and can request to be discharged against medical advice (AMA).

Quiz

1. You walk into the room and find the patient lying on the floor. What do you chart?

   a. Entered the room at 5:30 p.m. Pt fell out of bed on the floor left of the bed. Pt was alert, conscious, oriented. Left bed rail down. Right bed rail up.

   b. Entered the room at 5:30 p.m. Pt on the floor left of the bed. Pt was alert, conscious, oriented. Left bed rail down. Right bed rail up.

   c. Entered the room. Pt fell out of bed on the floor left of the bed. Pt was alert, conscious, oriented. Left bed rail down. Right bed rail up.

   d. Entered the room. Pt fell out of bed. Pt was alert, conscious, oriented. Left bed rail down. Right bed rail up.

2. You enter the room and see that the patient's intravenous line is disconnected from the patient's arm. The patient tells you, "I don't want this thing hooked up to me anymore." What do you chart?

   a. Entered room at 5:30 p.m. Saline lock not attached to the patient. Pt says, "I don't want this thing hooked up to me anymore."

   b. Entered room. Saline lock not attached to the patient.

   c. Entered room at 5:30 p.m. Saline lock not attached to the patient.

   d. Saline lock not attached to the patient.

3. After leaving the patient's room, the physician tells you that she is DNR. An hour later, the patient goes into cardiac arrest. The best response is to:

　a. Don't call a code.

　b. Call a code.

　c. Determine if the physician has written a DNR order.

　d. Call a slow code.

4. Your patient is scheduled to undergo an appendectomy. The physician ordered insertion of a urinary catheter. Before performing the procedure, you inform the patient of the physician's order. The patient refuses permission for you to perform the procedure. What is your best response?

　a. Perform the procedure because the surgical team is in the operating room waiting for the patient.

　b. Don't perform the procedure and then notify the physician that the patient refused the procedure.

　c. Explain the necessity of performing the procedure to the patient and then proceed to insert the catheter.

　d. Notify the Legal Department of the healthcare facility.

5. A physician writes a DNR order for your patient who is terminally ill with cancer. Forty-eight hours later the patient shows signs of severe respiratory distress. She is alert and oriented. She indicates that she wants to be placed on a respirator. What is the best response?

　a. Call the physician and prepare for her to be placed on the respirator.

　b. Tell her that her physician has written a DNR order.

　c. Notify the Legal Department of the healthcare facility.

　d. Begin cardiopulmonary resuscitation (CPR).

6. The patient is preparing to enter the operating room for routine removal of his gallbladder. He is drowsy from medication that was administered an hour ago. You noticed that the patient did not sign an informed consent for the operation. What is the best response?

　a. Proceed with the operation because the physician knows that the patient verbally agreed to the surgery.

　b. Have the patient sign the informed consent immediately.

　c. Notify the surgeon immediately.

　d. Ask the surgeon or another nurse to witness the patient's response after you ask the patient if he wants to proceed with the surgery.

7. You overhear a nursing assistant saying that she helped a patient back to bed after he slipped putting on his slippers. What is the best response?

   a. Report the nursing assistant to your supervisor.

   b. Write an incident report.

   c. Ask the nursing assistant to write an incident report.

   d. Thank the nursing assistant for helping the patient.

8. The patient arrives in the emergency department with pain in his lower right abdomen. The pain suddenly goes away. He refuses medical care and wants to leave the hospital so he can be at his brother's wedding. The nurse and the physician advise him not to leave because the sudden absence of pain can signify that his condition worsened. He still insists on leaving. What is the best response?

   a. Have the patient sign the discharge Against Medical Advice form and let him leave.

   b. Have the patient sign the discharge Against Medical Advice form. Before letting him leave, teach him how to recognize signs that his condition is worsening and where to go for immediate care.

   c. Don't let him go until he is treated.

   d. Keep explaining to him the risks involved with leaving the hospital.

9. The physician has written a DNR order for your terminally ill cancer patient. His family members are the only ones in the room when the patient becomes unconscious. Family members tell you that right before the patient became unconscious he said that he wanted everything done so he could live. What is the best response?

   a. Tell the family that the physician wrote a DNR order.

   b. Call the Legal Department of your facility.

   c. Remove the DNR order from the chart.

   b. Call another nurse into the room to witness the family's statement.

10. A 45-year-old man is being treated for gout. He is sleeping when his 21-year-old son arrives to visit. The son is concerned about his father's condition and demands to see his father's chart. The best response is?

    a. Explain that you are not permitted to do so because of patient confidentiality laws and reassure him that his father is receiving proper care.

    b. Show him the chart under your supervision.

    c. Show him the chart.

    d. Call security.

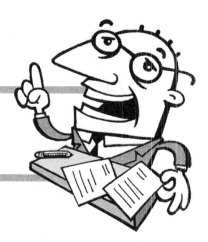

CHAPTER 3

Charting Medication and Normal Routines

No doubt, the first time you were required to update your patient's chart you probably stared in fear at the blank form in the chart. What should you write? This is a critical question to answer because your words become part of the patient's official record that will be used by other members of the healthcare team to decide the best course of treatment for the patient.

Furthermore, the patient's health insurer might base reimbursements to your healthcare facility according to what you write in the patient's chart. And medical and legal experts could scrutinize your writing years later should the patient's care result in litigation.

Charting must be thorough and complete, yet brief. Think of charting as writing a news report about the patient rather than the patient's life story. In this chapter, you'll learn how to chart the most frequent routines that you'll encounter as a staff nurse on a unit.

The MAR

The Medication Administration Record (MAR) is a working document that lists medications that are ordered for a patient and is used to document whether or not those medications were administered.

The design of an MAR differs among healthcare facilities; however, each has the same sections. These are:

- Patient Information (Figure 3-1): This includes the patient's name, identification number, room number, diagnosis, and allergies.

- Schedule Medications (Figure 3-2): These are medications that are given regularly to the patient to maintain a therapeutic level such as once a day for 7 days.

Unit	Patient's Name	Allergies		Primary Nurse
Med Surg	Susan Jones	None		Bob Marks
Room #				**Social Worker**
1601			**Age**	Roberta Johnson
		52		**Resident Physician**
			DOB	Dr. Anne Ford
		03/05/55		**Attending Physician**
				Dr. John Merk

Figure 3-1

Medication Administration Record										
Order Date Initials	Exp. Date Time	Medication-Dosage-Frequency Rt. Of Adm.	HR	4/1	4/2	4/3	4/4	4/5	4/6	

Figure 3-2

- Single Orders (Figure 3-3): These are medications that are administered once for an immediate effect such as epinephrine given stat for anaphylactic shock.
- PRN Medications (Figure 3-4): These are medications given as needed such as a nonsteroidal anti-inflammatory drug (NSAID) for pain relief.

Code		
O = Omitted	/ = Outdated	Cut = Discontinued
1 = Upper Outer Quadrant R Buttock	7 = Rt. Lateral Thigh	13 = Lt. Anterior Lateral Abdomen
2 = Upper Outer Quadrant L Buttock	8 = Lt. Lateral Thigh	14 = Rt. Posterior Lateral Abdomen
3 = Rt. Deltoid	9 = Rt. Ventroguteal Area	15 = Lt. Posterior Lateral Abdomen
4 = Lt. Deltoid	10 = Lt. Ventrogluteal Area	16 = Rt. Upper Outer Arm
5 = Rt. Mid Anterior Thigh	11 = Abdomen	17 = Lt. Upper Outer Arm
6 = Lt. Mid Anterior Thigh	12 = Rt. Anterior Lateral Abdomen	

Single Orders-Pre-operatives Stat-Meds						
Order Date Initials	Medication-Dosage-Route	Date Time	Adm. Time	Time Given	Site	Nurse Initial

Figure 3-3

PRN Medications								
Order Date Initials	Stop Date	Medication-Dosage-Frequency Rt. Of Adm.	PRN Medications-Doses Given					
			Date					
			Time					
			Init.					
			Site					
			Date					
			Time					
			Init.					
			Site					
			Date					
			Time					
			Init.					
			Site					

Figure 3-4

Full Signature	Title	Initial
Bob Marks	RN	BM
Mary Adams	RN	MA

Figure 3-5

- Signature (Figure 3-5): Each healthcare provider who administers a medication to the patient must be identified by full signature, title, and initials entered into the signature section of the MAR. Initials are then placed on the MAR alongside the medications that the healthcare provider administered to the patient.

CREATING A NEW MAR

A new MAR is created when the patient is admitted to the healthcare facility by the admissions staff or by the unit secretary, who enters general information about the patient on the MAR and places it into the Medication Administration Record section of the patient's chart.

Prescriptions, written by a physician for medication, are copied from the Medical Orders section of the patient's chart and entered into the appropriate section of the MAR using a process called taking off orders (see Taking Off Orders).

A licensed registered nurse (RN) is responsible for taking off orders, although it is generally the unit secretary who initially takes off an order, all orders are always reviewed and signed off by a registered nurse. The registered nurse is legally responsible for the accuracy in the transcribing of medical orders on the MAR.

INFORMATION ABOUT MEDICATION

The MAR is a time-saving tool because it contains information needed to administer medications to a patient, except for orders that are cancelled or have not been taken off as yet. It is for this reason that you must always review the latest medical orders prior to administering any medication.

For each medication, the MAR contains:

- Order date: This is the date that the physician ordered the medication.
- Expiration date: The order is no longer valid on or after the expiration date of the order.

- Medication name: This is usually the brand name of the medication.

- Dose: The amount of the medication the patient receives in a specified period of time.

- Frequency: The number of doses the patient receives.

- Route of administration: The route in which the medication is given to the patient.

- Site of administration: Where was the medication administered if medication was an injection?

- Date and time: The day and hour that the medication must be administered.

USING THE MAR

At the beginning of each shift, the primary nurse reviews the MAR and identifies medications scheduled to be administered to the patient during the shift. The primary nurse also reviews the patient's chart for any new orders or cancelled orders that were written since the MAR was last updated. These orders, if they exist, are then taken off by the primary nurse.

Hint Make a note of orders that are scheduled to expire at the end of the shift. Depending on the patient's condition and the nature of the order, you may want to ask the physician if the order should be renewed.

Next, each medication is located on the unit. Medications delivered regularly by the pharmacy are usually placed in the patient's drawer in the medical cabinet or in the medication room. Each is labeled with the patient's name, identification, and room number. It is important to locate medications at the beginning of the shift, thus allowing time to follow up with the pharmacy if the medication can't be found.

Before preparing to administer medication, one last check is made of the Medical Order section of the patient's chart to determine if the physician cancelled the order or prescribed new medication. This is an important step since in a busy unit the primary nurse may not have the opportunity to speak directly with the physician.

The MAR is updated once the medication is administered to the patient. Some healthcare facilities require the primary nurse to take the MAR into the patient's room when administering medication so that the MAR can be immediately updated, giving little room for error.

Other healthcare facilities require the primary nurse to update the MAR immediately upon returning to the nurse's station after administering the medication to the patient. This leaves room for error since the primary nurse can easily be distracted and fail to remember to update the MAR.

The MAR is updated using one of three methods depending on the order:

- Scheduled medication: Write your initials in the cells that corresponds to the date and time that the medication was ordered.
- Single orders: Write the date, time, site, and your initials.
- PRN: Enter the date, time, site, and your initials.

CAUTION *The nurse updates the MAR after administering medication, documenting that the patient received the ordered medication. Never do this before administering the medication.*

THE PRESCRIPTION

A prescription is an order for medication that is written on a prescription form if the patient is going to receive it after leaving the healthcare facility.

The physician must clearly specify in a prescription the medication and how it is to be administered. The prescription must contain the

- Name of the medication
- Dose
- Number of doses
- Route
- Frequency
- Start and end dates for administering

The actual time that the medication is administered is determined by the nurse when pulling down the order unless the physician otherwise specifies. For example, the physician may order that the medication be administered twice a day. The nurse determines this means 8 a.m. and 8 p.m. based on the healthcare facility's policy.

The physician's medication order may specify a condition must exist before the medication is given to the patient. For example, it is common for a physician to order different doses of insulin, called a sliding scale, based on the patient's serum glucose level. The nurse tests the patient's serum glucose and based on the results administers the desired number of units of insulin.

HINT *Some healthcare facilities place orders for insulin given on a sliding scale in the Medical Orders section of the patient's chart instead of the prescription section of the MAR.*

TIP For a patient being discharged, a prescription is written on a prescription form and placed into the Discharge section of the patient's chart. The nurse then gives the patient the prescription as part of the patient's discharge orders.

The KARDEX

The KARDEX is a quick reference document commonly used on a unit to provide the healthcare team with information about the patient brought together into one place and readily available without having to search through the patient's chart.

Each healthcare facility has its own form of a KARDEX. With the integration of a computer charting system, many facilities now have the capability of generating a computer-based KARDEX, although some still use cards stored in a flip chart or standard sheets of paper that are stored in a loose-leaf binder. Regardless of the form, all contain the same kind of information.

Information found on a KARDEX includes:

- Orders for diagnostic procedures and/or treatments (other than medications) (Figure 3-6): These are orders taken off the Medical Order section of the patient's chart for lab tests and procedures used to diagnose the patient. Each is listed along with the date it was ordered (a paper KARDEX may indicate the date it was completed). Note, however, that the computer-generated "kardex" is printed every day and updated with current orders only—listing as above; information regarding completion of the procedure or treatment would be handed off during a verbal, taped, or written "hand-off" report at the end of every shift.

- General Patient Information: Patient's name, room number, age, date of birth, allergies, diagnosis.

Patient KARDEX					
Date Ordered	Diagnostic Procedures	Date Done	Date Ordered	Vital Signs/Treatments	Expir. Date

Figure 3-6

- The Healthcare Team: The attending physician is listed here. On a paper KARDEX, other departments involved with the care may be listed; for example, physical therapy, occupational therapy, respiratory therapy. A computer-generated KARDEX may only list the attending physician; other departments will document involvement with care on the interdisciplinary progress record.
- Specialty Information. The medical team caring for patients on a specialty unit such as ICU, psychiatry, and cardiology need key information that otherwise would not be found on a general-purpose KARDEX. Therefore, healthcare facilities typically design specialty KARDEXs for these units.

Taking Off Orders

Medical orders written for medication, treatments, and diagnostic tests must be copied from the Medical Orders section of the patient's chart to the MAR and KARDEX. This process is called taking off orders. This is a critical process because failure to accurately transfer the order can have serious consequences for the patient.

Many healthcare facilities require an RN to take off orders; however, some healthcare facilities authorize trained staff such as a unit secretary to take off orders if reviewed and signed off by an RN.

Orders for medication contain most, but not all, the information that must be entered into an MAR. Physicians typically don't specify the exact time to administer scheduled medication. Instead physicians use medical abbreviations to indicate the number of doses to administer to the patient. For example, the physician will write "daily" on the prescription if the patient is to receive one dose per day.

The primary nurse is responsible for translating this into a medication schedule when taking off the order using the healthcare facility's policy as a guide. Some healthcare facilities require that medication ordered once a day be given at 10 a.m.

Orders for treatments and tests also typically lack specific times. The physician will write "upper GI series" and the test schedule with other departments in the healthcare facility and then update the KARDEX.

HOW TO TAKE OFF AN ORDER

Let's say that the physician wrote the following prescription:

Lasix 40 mg PO daily

KCl 20 mEq PO daily

The medications above are considered to be scheduled medications as they indicate that the patient will take them every day until the order expiration date, which is generally 7 days after the initial order is written.

In most systems, the health-care provider writes the order and flags the chart. This alerts the unit secretary that there is a new order written for the patient. In a computerized system, the order is directly entered into the computerized chart and the RN electronically signs off on the order.

The primary RN or the charge RN designee verifies the order for its accuracy in the computer. This verification is then seen by the pharmacist who will also verify the order, mark it as a verified order, fill it, and send the medication to the unit for the patient.

In a paper system, the same steps would be taken, and the verification by the RN is noted with his or her initials. A copy is sent to pharmacy and the pharmacist will verify the order, fill it, and send it back to the unit.

The nurse then takes off the order by writing it in the MAR as shown in Figure 3-7.

The physician might write a single order for medication such as:

Morphine sulfate 2 mg IVP now × 1

Medication Administration Record											
Order Date Initials	Exp. Date Time	Medication-Dosage-Frequency Rt. Of Adm.	HR	4/1	4/2	4/3	4/4	4/5	4/6	4/7
4/1 BM	4/7	Lasix 40 mg PO qd	1000							
4/1 BM	4/7	**Kcl 20 meq qd**	1000							

Figure 3-7

A single order is just that. The nurse can follow that order only once and the order expires. In a computer system, the nurse will enter the order, administer the medication, and chart it as given. The unit secretary can also enter this order, and then the system as above will follow for RN/pharmacist verification. In a paper system, the medication is written in the designated area for one time–only medications and the system above is followed. This is illustrated in Figure 3-8.

PRN is another type of prescription that the physician might write as:

Zofran 4 mg IVP q6h PRN for nausea

Acetaminophen 650 mg PO q6h PRN for temp >100.5

The system in place for taking off a PRN order would be the same as the system used for a one-time order and/or a scheduled medication. PRN orders are placed in the PRN area of the MAR as shown in Figure 3.9.

Treatment orders must also be taken off and placed in the KARDEX. Say that the physician ordered the following treatment and two medical tests.

Nebulizer Albuterol (2.5 mg/3mL) 2.5 mg/Ipratropium (0.5/2.5 mg) 0.5 mg q4 & q2 PRN for audible wheezing

MRI Brain with contrast, Indications: R/O meningitis

MRI ABD WO Contrast, organ to be scanned, Indications R/O biliary mass

Code		
O = Omitted	/ = Outdated	Cut = Discontinued
1 = Upper Outer Quadrant R Buttock	7 = Rt. Lateral Thigh	13 = Lt. Anterior Lateral Abdomen
2 = Upper Outer Quadrant L Buttock	8 = Lt. Lateral Thigh	14 = Rt. Posterior Lateral Abdomen
3 = Rt. Deltoid	9 = Rt. Ventroguteal Area	15 = Lt. Posterior Lateral Abdomen
4 = Lt. Deltoid	10 = Lt. Ventrogluteal Area	16 = Rt. Upper Outer Arm
5 = Rt. Mid Anterior Thigh	11 = Abdomen	17 = Lt. Upper Outer Arm
6 = Lt. Mid Anterior Thigh	12 = Rt. Anterior Lateral Abdomen	

Single Orders-Pre-operatives Stat-Meds						
Order Date Initials	Medication-Dosage-Route	Date Time	Adm. Time	Time Given	Site	Nurse Initial
4/1 BM	MS 2 mg IVP now one time	4/1 1500		1515	IV	BM

Figure 3-8

PRN Medications										
Order Date Initials	**Stop Date**	**Medication-Dosage-Frequency Rt. Of Adm.**		**PRN Medications-Doses Given**						
4/1	4/7	Zofran 4 mg IVP PRN for nausea	Date	4/1						
			Time	08:00						
BM			Init.	BM						
			Site	IV						
4/1	4/7	Acetaminophen 650 mg PO q6h PRN for temp > 100.5	Date	4/1						
			Time	1015						
BM			Init.	BM						
			Site	IV						
			Date							
			Time							
			Init.							
			Site							

Figure 3-9

Treatment orders and medical orders are both handled the same way, and similar to any medication order, following the system check between unit secretary and RN. Once the orders are verified, they will appear on a computer-generated KARDEX with the date of order; they will appear on a paper KARDEX with a date of order and a date of completion when appropriate. This is shown in Figure 3-10.

Patient KARDEX						
Date Ordered	**Diagnostic Procedures**	**Date Done**	**Date Ordered**	**Vital Signs/Treatments**	**Expir. Date**
4/1	MRI Brain with contrast	4/2	4/1	Nebulizer Albuterol 2.5 mg/ Ipratropium 0.5 mg q4H & q2h prn for audible wheezing	4/7
4/3	MRI ABD w/o contrast	4/3			

Figure 3-10

Avoid Common Errors When Using the MAR and KARDEX

Errors can occur when taking off orders and recording when medication is administered to a patient resulting in overmedicating or undermedicating the patient or administering incorrect medication.

Steps can be taken to assure that the most common of these errors is avoided. Here is what you need to do:

- Use abbreviations that are approved by JCAHO (Joint Commission on Accreditation of Healthcare Organizations) and adopted by your healthcare facility. For example, all healthcare facilities require that "daily" replace the abbreviation OD and "every other day" be used in place of QOD. Always write the full word if you are unsure of the abbreviation to write. Refer to your facility's Dangerous Abbreviations policy for clarification.

- JCAHO requires writing numbers by dropping the zero following a decimal if the dose is a whole number and use a zero to the left of the decimal if the dose is a fraction. Write 1 mg instead of 1.0 mg and 0.5 mg instead of .5 mg.

- Be sure that your full name, title, and initials appear on the MAR and KARDEX before initializing that you administered medication or performed a procedure or diagnostic test.

- Update the MAR immediately after you administer medication to a patient.

- Write legibly on all documents. Assume no one else can read your handwriting is so make whatever your write, easy to read.

- Circle any medication that wasn't administered and write the reason why it was omitted in the MAR or in the Nurse Progress Notes if there isn't sufficient space to include comments in the MAR. (Check your healthcare facility's policy for further instruction.)

- Write in the MAR the reason for administering PRN medication.

- Note the assessment results on the MAR if particular assessments must be made before administering medication (i.e., the patient's blood pressure before administering blood pressure medication).

HINT *If the patient refuses medication, write the patient's own words in quotations in the MAR and/or in the Nurse Progress Notes and other documents required by your healthcare facility.*

Charting Narcotics

Healthcare facilities require additional documentation for opioids. Many healthcare facilities use a computer-controlled cabinet (PYXIS) located in the medication room to dispense opioids. The computer automatically documents dispensing the medication, which includes the medication, dose, patient, and the nurse who retrieved the medication.

Other healthcare facilities who don't use a computer-controlled cabinet manually document the inventory of opioids within the locked area of the medication room by using the opioids inventory control form.

At the beginning of each shift, one RN from the offgoing shift and an RN from the oncoming shift count the number of opioids in the medication room and compare the total to the current balance on the opioids inventory control form. Any difference is reported to the nursing supervisor.

During the shift, the patient's primary nurse records the name, dose, and patient's identifier on the opioids inventory control form and signs the form when preparing to administer the opioid to a patient. This amount is deducted from the current balance and a new current balance is entered on the opioids inventory control form.

CAUTION *Any opioid that is discarded must be witnessed by an RN. Both the primary nurse and the witness must sign the opioids inventory control form stating the reason for discarding the medication.*

IV Administration

IV medications are documented on an IV administration form that is sometimes combined with a fluid intake and output form (Figure 3-11). Additional information is entered into the Nurse Progress Notes. Every aspect of administering the IV should be documented.

Progress Notes
08:30 Heparin lock Lt wrist intact, no redness or swelling noted
10:30 Heparin lock Lt wrist red, tender to touch, bleeding at site
13:00 Heparin lock Lt wrist phlebitis noted
15:30 Heparin lock Lt wrist infiltrated, cool to touch, painful to touch, disrupted flow
rate No blood return

Figure 3-11

Here is information that you need to provide:

- Date and time when administration began.
- Name of medication or blood product given to the patient.
- Type and location of the IV lock.
- Complications such as number of attempts to insert the lock and who inserted the lock.
- The amount of IV fluid hung.
- The rate of flow of the IV.
- Whether or not gravity feed or a pump is used.

At least each shift, you'll need to examine the IV site and assess the IV flow. You'll need to document:

- The condition of the IV site (see Figure 3-11).
- Flushing the lock with saline or heparin solution.
- The date, time, and the amount of fluid left in the bag if you stop and remove the IV.
- The amount of fluid left in the bag if you change bags and the amount of fluid and rate of flow if you hang a new bag.
- The date, time, type, and location of the IV lock if you changed the location of the IV lock.

Intake and Output Flow Chart

It is important for a physician to know the amount of fluids a patient receives and the amount of fluids that the patient excretes in a 24-hour period depending on the nature of the patient's condition. This is commonly referred to as the patient's intake and output and is recorded on the Intake and Output form (Figures 3-12 and 3-13).

Intake includes liquids that the patient

- Takes my mouth (meals)
- Through gastrostomy (PEG) feeding tubes
- Through nasogastric feeding tubes
- IV fluids
- Blood or its components

IV Administration				INTAKE				
Time	IV Fluid/Blood Products	Rate	CC's Hung/LIB	IV CC's Rec'd	PO	Tube Feed	NG/GI IRRIG	Hourly Running Total
00:00								
01:00								
02:00								
03:00								
04:00								
05:00								
06:00								
07:00								
Total								
08:00								
09:00								
10:00								
11:00								
12:00								
13:00								
14:00								
15:00								
Total								
16:00								
17:00								
18:00								
19:00								
20:00								
21:00								
22:00								
23:00								
Total								
				Total Intake, 24 HRS:				

Figure 3-12

- Liquid medication
- Fluids used to flush tubes

Output includes:

- Urine
- Diarrhea
- Vomitus
- Gastric suction
- Wound drainage and type of drain

The amount of fluid is entered in the appropriate cell in the Input and Output form according to the time and nature of the fluid. It is important to record fluids in milliliters, although some healthcare facilities might use centimeters as the unit of measurement. This means that you will need to convert household measurements to milliliters (mL) before recording it (Table 3-1).

Output						
Time	NG/GI	STOOL	MESIS	URINE	OTHER	Hourly Running Total
00:00						
01:00						
02:00						
03:00						
04:00						
05:00						
06:00						
07:00						
Total						
08:00						
09:00						
10:00						
11:00						
12:00						
13:00						
14:00						
15:00						
Total						
16:00						
17:00						
18:00						
19:00						
20:00						
21:00						
22:00						
23:00						
Total						
				Total Output, 24 HRS:		

Figure 3-13

Most fluid taken by the patient is premeasured, making it straightforward to record the volume on the Intake and Output form. Likewise, most fluid excreted by the patient can be easily measured using an appropriate device. However, you will be required to measure fluid intake and output that isn't premeasured or is difficult to measure.

Table 3-1 Converting Common Household Measurements

Household Measurement	Milliliter Equivalent
1 ounce	30 mL
1 teaspoon	5 mL
1 tablespoon	15 mL

For example, ice chips would be written as ice chips or approximate as sips—10 mL and so forth; Jell-O or gelatin, measured by milliliters—an approximate amount based on the container size of the product.

AVOIDING COMMON MISTAKES

Here are common errors that occur when measuring intake and output. Knowing these will help you avoid them.

Intake

- The patient eats snacks and drinks juice or soft drinks without the knowledge of the nurse
- Not including IV push medication
- Failing to record IV piggybacks
- Flushing tubes
- Fluids taken while the patient undergoes tests outside of the unit
- Fluids swallowed such as liquid medication

Output

- The patient who has bathroom privileges voids and fails to notify the nurse
- Bleeding
- Incontinence

Transferring a Patient

Every time a patient is moved from one unit to another, you must document the transfer in the nurse's notes. The nurse's notes contain pertinent information that describes the transfer for both the current unit and the receiving unit. A patient can be transferred to another unit permanently or can be transferred to another department temporarily. Regardless of where the patient is going, documentation must indicate that the patient has left the unit.

Some healthcare facilities may use separate documentation to indicate information about the patient's transfer. Separate documentation may be used when the patient is leaving with a transporter or unlicensed person and it will indicate where the patient is going and why he or she is going off the unit.

The general information that would be included is:

- Date and time of the transfer
- Name of the current unit
- Name of the receiving unit

The nurse's notes also describe the condition of the patient when the patient left the unit and the condition of the patient when the patient arrived at the new unit. Also document the reason for the transfer. Any change in the patient's condition that occurs during the transfer is also noted.

Be sure to include:

- Description of any wounds
- Location of heparin locks
- Description of medical devices that are connected to the patient during the transfer
- Vital signs
- Allergies
- Advance directives
- Significant procedures or events involving the patient
- The patient's ability to communicate
- Names of staff who accompanied the patient during the transfer

DOCUMENTING A TRANSFER

The nurse must assess the patient before the patient is transferred and document this assessment in the nurse's notes. Only a stable patient should leave the unit with an unlicensed person.

An unstable patient should not be transferred unless the patient is accompanied by an RN and is constantly being monitored with an electrocardiogram or other appropriate equipment. This should be noted in the nurse's notes.

The patency of oxygen, IV, and other forms of ongoing treatment must be assessed and noted in the nurse's notes before the patient leaves the unit.

Precautions when transferring: The transfer RN needs to assess the patient prior to transfer.

GIVING A CHARGE REPORT

The nurse who is taking over primary care for the patient in the receiving unit must be brought up-to-date on the patient's status. This is accomplished when the patient's current primary nurse gives the Charge Report.

The Charge Report is verbal documentation of the patient's condition. It can be given over the telephone before the patient arrives on the unit or in person if the primary nurse accompanies the patient to the new unit.

The transfer of a patient isn't complete until the Charge Report is given to the nurse who is accepting primary care for the patient. The Charge Report should follow JCAHO standards for hand-off communications. This standard is easy to follow if you remember the acronym ISBAR.

Here is the information that you need to provide the other nurse:

- Introduction: Identify yourself and the patient.
- Situation: Tell the nurse the patient's chief complaint/diagnosis. Also include significant events and the patient's needs and problems.
- Background: Give a synopsis of the patient's treatment, vital signs, pain level, complaints, and assessment changes.
- Assessment: Provide the nurse with a conclusion about the patient's situation, overall body systems involved, and if the patient is in a life-threatening situation.
- Recommendation: Tells the nurse what you feel would be helpful to him/ her such as medications and tests scheduled for the patient, if the patient will be transferred again, and clarify all orders.

Another acronym that is handy to remember when giving a transfer or end-of-shift report is I-PASS-THE-BATON. This is:

- Introduction: Introduce yourself.
- Patient: Identify the patient.
- Assessment: Chief complaint/diagnosis, vital signs/symptoms.
- Situation: Code status/circumstances/recent changes/response to treatment/ current status.

- Safety concerns: Critical labs/reports/allergies/alerts—falls, isolation, and so forth.
- Background: Comorbidities/family history, current medications, previous episodes.
- Actions: What actions have been taken or required and why?
- Timing: What is the priority for the actions?
- Ownership: Who is managing this patient? Attending? Consults?
- Next: What are the plans for this patient?

Summary

Charts are used by the patient's healthcare team, healthcare insurer, and others involved in the patient's well-being to document facts related to the patient's health and treatment. *Charting* is the term used to describe documenting patient information and must be thorough, complete, and yet brief.

There are several kinds of documentation used in routine patient care:

- The Medication Administration Record (MAR) is used to document whether or not medications were administered to the patient.
- The KARDEX is a quick-reference document that brings together information about the patient into one place without having to search through the patient's chart.
- Opioids Inventory Control Form is used to document the inventory of opioids within the locked area of the medication room.
- Intake and Output Form is used to document the amount of fluids a patient receives and the amount of fluids that the patient excretes in a 24-hour period.
- The Transfer Form is used to document when a patient is transferred to another unit

Quiz

1. What is the best form used to record the amount of IV fluid that was given to a patient?
   a. Transfer Form
   b. Intake and Output Form

c. Progress Notes

   d. KARDEX

2. The purpose of giving a report to the new primary nurse is to

   a. Provide a complete and thorough history of the patient.

   b. Quickly bring the nurse up-to-date on the patient's status.

   c. Give a detailed status of all the patient's medical tests.

   d. Introduce the nurse to the patient's preferences.

3. A common error in recording a patient's intake and output is not including

   a. A heparin flush

   b. Washing hair

   c. Discarded medication

   d. Time-release capsule

4. The medical laboratory never has to be informed of medication given to the patient immediately prior to taking a blood sample.

   a. True

   b. False

5. Transferring medical orders to the KARDEX is called taking off orders

   a. True

   b. False

6. The best way to avoid errors when updating the MAR is to

   a. Use abbreviations adopted by your healthcare facility

   b. Update the MAR immediately after you administer medication to a patient

   c. Drop the zero following the decimal

   d. All of the above

7. Always make note of orders that are scheduled to expire at the end of the shift.

   a. True

   b. False

8. Medications that are given regularly to the patient to maintain a therapeutic level such as once a day for 7 days are documented as

   a. Double Order

   b. PRN

c. Single Orders

    d. Schedule Medication

9. Always circle any medication that wasn't administered and write the reason why it was omitted in the MAR

    a. True

    b. False

10. At the beginning of the shift, balance the Opioid Inventory Control Form with a nurse from the outgoing shift

    a. True

    b. False

CHAPTER 4

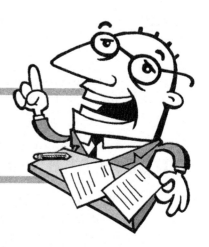

Patient Care Plans

A patient who is admitted to a healthcare facility receives care from a healthcare team that is coordinated by the patient's primary physician. The team consists of primary nurses (one for each shift), a nurse manager or director, nursing assistants, and specialists in a variety of disciplines depending on the patient's needs.

The team works from an interdisciplinary patient care plan—a kind of playbook—used to guide the healthcare team through diagnostic tests, medical procedures, and routines that assure that the patient receives the best possible care.

There are many forms of care plans, all of which contain the same key information to direct the healthcare team: the patient's problem, interventions to address each problem, and the expected outcome or goal of these interventions. At the foundation of any care plan is the nursing process; therefore evaluation is always part of the plan. A student care plan will provide a column for the evaluation of the intervention. The evaluation of an intervention on an institutional plan of care becomes part of the charting process, which includes a comprehensive narrative note written by the nurse when the intervention has not been successful. At that point, the nurse will revise the intervention on the care plan by changing some of the criteria, and hopefully arriving at the expected outcome.

In this chapter, you'll learn how to write a care plan and use a care plan as a tool for caring for the patient.

Purpose of a Care Plan

Think of a care plan as a road map of a patient's healthcare. It contains the patient's healthcare problems that were identified when the patient was assessed and it contains actions for the healthcare team to take to minimize or resolve those problems. Each action must be based on a scientific rationale, have a measurable outcome, and be patient specific. That is, the action is proven to work and the healthcare team can measure if the action did minimize or resolve the patient's problem.

For example, a patient on total bed rest is at risk for decubitus ulcers (bed sores). The healthcare team will turn the position of the patient in bed every 2 hours. It has been proven that turning the position of the patient frequently will reduce the risk for decubitus ulcers, which is why this action is taken. Examining the patient for decubitus ulcers at the beginning of each shift determines if repositioning the patient every 2 hours prevented decubitus ulcers.

DEFINING A PROBLEM

The healthcare team assesses the signs and symptoms presented by the patient to determine the patient's problems. Each problem is described as a nursing diagnosis. A nursing diagnosis is a standardized statement defined by a recognized body such as the North American Nursing Diagnosis Association (NANDA). The problem is described in the nursing plan using the nursing diagnosis.

There are many styles of care plans. There are student care plans and institutional care plans. For a student-type care plan, one will usually use the PES format to identify a problem. The PES format has three components:

P is the problem stated as a nursing diagnosis

E is the etiology-origin of the problem

S is the sign/symptoms that lead the healthcare team to choose this nursing diagnosis

The PES format is written as:

P: nursing diagnosis from the NANDA list of nursing diagnosis

E: Related to; specify the patient's condition that is related to this problem

S: As evidence by list signs/symptoms

Let's say that the patient who is being treated for deep tissue laceration of the left inferior calf is experiencing pain. Here is one way to describe this problem using the PES format:

P: Acute pain

E: Related to deep tissue laceration of the left inferior calf

S: As evidenced by the patient reporting a pain level 8 on a scale of 0–10

SETTING GOALS

Goals are set for each patient problem. A goal is a measurable outcome that is expected after the healthcare team performs the action. The number of goals defined depends on the nature of the patient's problem.

Each goal is assessed after the action is performed to determine if the desired result was achieved. The assessment is made using a standard measurement, which many times involves the patient reporting a condition or performing a behavior.

Here are a few goals for the patient with a deep tissue laceration. It is customary to number each goal.

1. Patient will report an acceptable pain level on a scale of 0–10.

2. Patient will report that the pain management regimen relieves pain to satisfactory level with acceptable and manageable side effects.

3. Patient will perform activities of recovery with reported acceptable level of pain.

HINT *A measurement can be subjective or objective. For example, measuring pain is subjective, based on the patient's definition of pain. A temperature of 100°F is objective and is not influenced by interpretation. Both subjective and objective measurements can be used to set goals.*

PLANNING ACTION

An action is something done to achieve goals that were set for the patient with regard to the nursing diagnosis. Just as goals are related to the patient's problem, actions are related to goals. Each goal could have one or more actions. Likewise, an action can achieve one or more goals. It all depends on the goal and action.

Each action typically begins with a verb such as assess, assist, explain, and teach and is followed by the description of the action. Here are a few actions for the patient with a deep tissue laceration. It is customary to number each action.

1. Assess the patient's pain level every 2 hours and PRN (as needed) using the scale of 0 to 10.

2. Teach patient to use stabilizing equipment or supportive measures when moving.

3. Assist patient with ADLs (activities of daily living) (use of bedpan) as needed to manage pain level.

4. Teach patient the myths and facts regarding physical/psychological addiction to narcotics.

5. Teach the patient to request pain medication before pain is severe.

SCIENTIFIC RATIONALE

There must be a scientific basis for each action. The scientific basis is usually a recognized standard of practice that is documented in a healthcare facilities policy, in an authoritative textbook, or published elsewhere.

Some nursing schools require that students include the scientific rationale in the care plan because instructors want to follow the student's thinking process for selecting an action. An institutional care plan will not include a scientific rationale for interventions. It is common that healthcare facilities standardize care plans according to typical patient profiles. Goals, actions, and other components of the care plan are predefined based on scientific rational. And they can be modified as needed to address the needs of the patient.

Student care plans generally require that each action have a scientific rationale. The scientific rationale is a sentence or paragraph that justifies the action followed by a reference. Rationales are numbered according to the number of the corresponding action.

Here are scientific rationales for actions for the patient with a deep tissue laceration:

1. The patient's verbalization of pain on a scale of 0 to 10 determines the effectiveness of pain medication administered to the patient. (Mosby's Medical-Surgical Nursing, page 138, by Paulette D. Rollant and Deborah A. Ennis **ISBN-10:** 0323011772.)

2. Supporting an injured leg reduces pressure on the wound and reduces pain to the patient. (Fundamentals of Nursing Potter, page 1483, by Patricia A. Potter and Anne Griffin Perry **ISBN-10:** 0323054234.)

3. Positioning a bedpan can be extremely uncomfortable. The nurse should help position the patient comfortably and support wound areas. (Fundamentals of Nursing Potter, page 1395, by Patricia A. Potter and Anne Griffin Perry **ISBN-10:** 0323054234.)

4. The patient may withhold self-medication for fear of developing addiction to pain medication. (Mosby's Medical-Surgical Nursing, page 154 by Paulette D. Rollant and Deborah A. Ennis **ISBN-10:** 0323011772.)

5. Treatment for pain requires that pain medication be given before pain occurs. (Mosby's Medical-Surgical Nursing, page 140 by Paulette D. Rollant and Deborah A. Ennis **ISBN-10:** 0323011772.)

EVALUATING THE OUTCOME

Were goals for the patient reached? That's the question answered in the evaluation portion of the student care plan. Every action is assessed to determine its impact on the patient and whether or not the goal was achieved.

The impact is described in a sentence or paragraph that usually begins with *The Patient* followed by an explanation of how the patient reacted to the action and if the goal associated with the action was reached.

Each evaluation is numbered to correspond with the goal.

Here are evaluations for the patient with a deep tissue laceration:

1. The patient reported a pain level of 8 on a scale of 0 to 10 when moving his left calf 20 minutes after the pain medication dose peaked.

2. The patient demonstrated correct use of the leg immobilizer prior to moving self out of bed.

3. The patient called the nurse for assistance when requiring a bedpan .

4. Patient verbalized understanding that requesting pain medication frequently will not lead to addiction.

5. Patient successfully anticipated pain and used the call button to ask the nurse for PRN medication. He frequently reports a pain level of 2 (0–10).

HINT *Goals are not always 100 percent achieved. The level of achievement is indicated in the evaluation. Also, an outcome may not be observed for a number of reasons. In these cases, write "not observed."*

Categories of Nursing Diagnosis

There are five categories of nursing diagnosis (NANDA). Each category contains a nursing diagnosis that can easily be mapped to the condition of the patient. The categories are:

- Actual Diagnosis focuses on the patients' health problem such as *acute pain.*

- Risk Diagnosis consists of potential problems that the patient is at risk for developing and begins with *risk for* such as risk for injury.

- Possible Diagnosis consists of problems that the patient may have, but there is insufficient information of it in the diagnosis. This begins with *possible* such as fluid volume excess.

- Syndrome Diagnosis is a problem that consists of a cluster of other diagnoses such as *chronic pain.*

- Wellness Diagnosis cosists of problems that could arise because of the patients' ill health and usually begins with, for example, *potential for.*

Care Plan Formats

There are many formats used for a care plan. All serve as a guide for providing care to the patient. They differ in the format style and the kind of information contained in the care plan. Your school or healthcare facility determines the best care plan format for their patients.

In this chapter, we'll discuss two care plan formats. The first is a comprehensive style that is similar to care plans students are required to create in nursing schools, generally referred to as a student care plan. The second type of care plan is referred to as an institutional care plan, or a care map. A care map is a comprehensive, interdisciplinary plan of care for a patient that includes a care plan utilizing the nursing process and identifying the nursing diagnosis, the interventions, and the expected outcomes for the patient. The care map will also include tools and keys that help to identify all of the care delivered for the patient in a 24-hour period. The care map, as an interdisciplinary tool, is designed for use by nurses and all members of the healthcare team.

NURSING CARE PLAN

The nursing care plan used by some nursing schools consists of six columns, although this will vary from school to school. Keep in mind, however, that prior to the columns, your school's care plan has asked you to provide a comprehensive assessment and has provided you with space for this. The assessment section in a student care plan will reflect the same information that a nurse would find in an institutional chart. That information consists of the following: admission data base; history and physical, which includes current and past medical and surgical history and results of the most current physical examination findings; social history; laboratory results data; diagnostic data; medication history.

In a student care plan, the first column is typically the assessment column for the identified problem. In other words, this column reflects the supporting data or the defining characteristics that lead you to the formation of the nursing diagnosis or the patient's problem (stating one problem at a time). For instance, your assessment data or defining characteristics for the diagnosis or problem of pain might include information such as pain level, medications ordered for treatment, and statements made by the patient that describe the pain level (Figure 4-1).

The next two columns (Figure 4-2) define the patient's problem (see Defining a Problem) and setting goals for the treatment (see Setting Goals). These columns are followed by three additional columns (Figure 4-3) that specify planning (see Planning Action), scientific rationales (see Scientific Rationale), and evaluating the intervention (see Evaluating the Outcome) taken by the medical team to address the patient's problem.

ASSESSMENT

(Defining Characteristics-Supporting Data)

- Pain level 8/10
- Using PCA Morphine pump
  continually
- Grimaces with any movement
- States "Pain is unbearable"

Figure 4-1

DIAGNOSIS Problem, etiology, symptoms	**GOALS**
P: Acute pain	Patient will report an acceptable pain level on a scale of 0–10.
E: Related to deep tissue laceration left inferior calf	Patient will report that pain management regimen relieves pain to satisfactory level with acceptable and manageable side effects.
S: As evidence by the patient report, a pain level 8 on a scale of 0–10	Patient will perform activities of recovery with reported acceptable level of pain.

Figure 4-2

PLANNING Interventions	SCIENTIFIC RATIONALES	EVALUATION
1. Assess the patient's pain level every two hours and PRN using the scale of 0–10	1. The patient's verbalization of pain on a scale of 0–10 determines the effectiveness of pain medication administered to the patient (Mosby's *Medical-Surgical Nursing*, page 138).	1. The patient reported a pain level of 8 on a scale of 0–10 when moving in left calf 20 minutes after the pain medication dose peaked.
2. Teach the patient to use stabilizing equipment or supporting measures when moving	2. Supporting an injured leg reduces pressure on the wound and reduces pain to the patient (*Fundamentals of Nursing*, Potter, page 1483).	2. The patient demonstrated correct use of the leg immobilizer prior to moving self out of bed.
3. Assist patient with ADLs to help manage pain level	3. Positioning a bedpan can be extremely uncomfortable. The nurse should help position clients comfortably and support wound areas (*Fundamentals of Nursing*, Potter, page 1395).	3. The patient called the nurse for assistance each time he felt a BM; however, he did not have a BM while under the nurse's care.
4. Teach patient myths/facts regarding: physical/psychological addiction to narcotics	4. The patient may withhold self-medication for fear of developing addiction to pain medication (Mosby's *Medical-Surgical Nursing*, page 154).	4. Patient verbalized that requesting pain medication frequently will not lead to addiction.
5. Teach patient to request pain medication before pain is severe	5. Treatment for pain requires that pain medication be given before pain occurs (Mosby's *Medical-Surgical Nursing*, page 140).	5. Patient successfully anticipated pain and used the call button to ask the nurse for PRN medication. He frequently reports a pain level of 2 (0–10).

Figure 4-3

Patient Problem	Expected Outcome	Nursing Orders
Respiratory: Risk for aspiration pneumonia as indicated by a. Pseudobulbar symptoms b. Bedridden	Normal respiration patterns No congestion Afebrile	1. Position the patient upright during feeding 2. Blenderized food 3. Feed the patient small portions 4. Deep breathing and coughing exercise q4h during waking hours

Figure 4-4

Figure 4-4 suggests another style of care plan where the plan is put together in three columns instead of six. This can resemble some student care plans or may be seen as an institutional care plan part of the care map (see Interdisciplinary Care Plans).

INTERDISCIPLINARY CARE PLAN

Interdisciplinary care plans, called care maps, are used by most healthcare institutions to provide continuity of care given by members of the patient's healthcare team to the patient, and also provide a uniformed approach to identifying the patient's needs, treatment, and expected outcomes. They are usually initiated by nursing team, and other team members will address issues on the care map as indicated. The interdisciplinary care map is really a combination of a care plan and the various documentation/charting tools that nursing and other health team members use to document the care. The tools will also include the admission database tool; so remember that this tool serves as the comprehensive assessment tool for the care plan using the nursing process as a foundation. Keep in mind that the format of the care plan portion of the care map may look similar to a student care plan in that it may use a columnar format as shown Figure 4-4. Regardless of the format used to indicate the patient's problems or Nursing Diagnoses, this (care plan) care map is a comprehensive picture of all problems identified for this patient for this hospitalization; a student care plan is a modified version of this, as a student care plan will generally only address one or two of the identified problems or nursing diagnoses.

Typically, a care map is divided into categories of patient care:

Nutrition

Assessment and Treatment

Teaching and Psychosocial

Specimens and Diagnostics

Safety and Activity

Discharge Plan

Each category contains interventions that are commonly performed by the healthcare team. Alongside each intervention is a box for day, evening, and night shifts to initial after the intervention is performed.

Nutrition

The nutrition category (Figure 4-5) contains a description of the patient's diet as one of the standard hospital diets as ordered by the physician. Table 4-1 contains diets commonly used in hospitals.

Also listed is the percentage of breakfast, lunch, and dinner consumed by the patient. The percentage is a rough estimate by the patient's primary nurse based on observation and not what the patient reports. The patient may report not eating very much and yet consumed 75% of his meal.

	D	E	N
Diet: REG	AB		
Diet Consumed:			
Breakfast 80%	AB		
Lunch 50%	AB		
Dinner 100%	AB		
Enteral Feedings: 50 mL/hr SUSTACAL	AB		
Parenteral feedings: TPN/Lipids			
Daily Weight 150 lb–standing scale			

Figure 4-5

Table 4-1   Common Hospital Diets

Diet	Description
Low residue	No fiber. No cellulose
High residue	Fiber, cellulose, cabbage, broccoli, apples, brown breads
Low fat	No saturated fat
Full liquid	All liquids, soft-oiled eggs (this is mechanically soft), custard
Clear liquid	Water, tea. No milk.
Sodium restricted	2000 mg; mild 1500–3000 mg; modest 500–1500 mg; severe 500 mg
Ulcer diet	No tea, no coffee, no raw foods, no hot foods, no cold foods
Gluten- free diet (BROW)	No barley, no rye, no oats, no wheat
Diabetic diet	1200, 1400, 1500, 1600, 2000, or 2200 calorie

There is also a subcategory for enteral feedings and parenteral feedings, which are based on medical orders. The nurse will document the type or name of the supplement the patient is receiving based on the medical order and the rate at which the supplement is administered.

The nutrition section has space to include the patient's daily weight. It is best to weight the patient at the same time each day using the same scale and having the patient dressed in the same attire. Weights are often done at the end of the night shift by the nursing assistant. Generally, the person charting the weight will indicate the scale used somewhere on the document—standing scale, bed scale, chair scale. One may also refer to the scale by the brand or company name. Weights will be documented either by kilograms or pounds, which is based on the hospital policy.

Assessment and Treatment

An interdisciplinary care plan has a section (Figure 4-6) that identifies standard assessments and treatment that most patients are expected to receive while admitted to a unit. Assessment and treatment reflect the specialty of the unit.

	D	E	N
Cardiac Monitor	AB		
Vital signs q __4_ hrs	AB		
I & O q __8_ hrs	AB		
D/C Foley			
O₂ Therapy : 3 LITERS NC	AB		
O₂ Sat q __8_ hrs	AB		
Incentive spirometry q 1 hr, while awake	AB		
C&DB q 1 hr. while awake	AB		
IV fluids as ordered	AB		
D/C IV _____ change to PIID			
Dressing change q _24__ hrs			
Tubes and Drains: Type: _____			
Pain Management: PO _____ IM PRN _____ PCA _____ Epidural _____ Continuous IV Infusion _____	AB		
DVT Prophy Laxis: Thigh/Knee High TEDS	AB		
Hygiene & Comfort	AB		
Peripheral IV Therapy	AB		
Pressure Ulcer Prevention	AB		
Respiratory Care	AB		

Figure 4-6

Each day every shift uses the same plan to document the required assessments and treatment. This assures continuity of care among shifts. Each nurse initials the assessment or treatment indicating that it was performed.

HINT *There is no universal key or format that all hospitals or institutions use for documenting purposes. Paperwork for each facility is designed and approved by administrative/nursing education personnel, using the standards set forth by accrediting bodies for that institution. However, the trend in most forms is to minimize writing/documentation for the nursing team. Generally, a normal response by a patient in any category is usually indicated by a check mark or a caregiver's initials. An abnormal response may be indicated by a circle, a time, and an initial, followed by a comprehensive narrative description of the abnormal response.*

Here are the standard assessments and treatments that you might find in a surgical unit:

- Vital signs at an interval specified by the physician
- Oxygen therapy at a specified rate and delivery method according to physician orders
- Monitoring oxygen saturation at an interval specified by the physician
- Administering the incentive spirometry every waking hour
- Cough and deep breath exercises every waking hour
- A description of IV fluids according to medical orders including the status of the IV site
- Intervals for assessing the site of any wounds and dressing changes
- Identifying drains and assessing the drainage
- Monitoring input and output
- The date a Foley catheter was inserted and the size of the catheter
- The date that the Foley catheter was discontinued
- A description of pain medication and assessing its effectiveness
- Orders for treatment that prevents deep vein thrombosis
- Treatment for preventing pressure ulcer

Teaching and Psychosocial

The teaching and psychosocial section of an interdisciplinary care plan focuses on the teaching needs of the patient and the family and/or significant others involved in the care. Teaching is the critical part of the discharge plan and begins on the day of admission. The goal of teaching is to prepare the patient for the discharge from the current level of medical care to home and/or a different level of care. The nurse provides the patient and others with comprehensive information that will facilitate the patient's ability to be cared for once outside the current medical facility.

Each shift, the primary nurse documents any new information given to the patient. The nurse indicates the topic taught, the method used for teaching, any barriers to teaching that may exist, and the patient's response to the teaching. For example, the nurse may teach the newly diagnosed Spanish-speaking patient with diabetes how to check a blood sugar. Documentation will include the equipment used to teach the skill, the method used to overcome the language barrier, and the patient's ability to demonstrate the skill learned to the nurse. Most care maps have a table/key designed to address the criteria; the nurse will also include a narrative note to describe the intervention. The care plan portion of the care map will also include the nursing diagnosis (problem) of knowledge deficit suggesting that problem. The nurse is expected to teach the patients all aspects of their care; thus relieving any anxiety that the patient may have regarding the diagnosis and the discharge plan. Other examples of topics discussed for teaching include medications (action, frequency, side effects, medication interactions), dressing changes, diet changes, and/or lifestyle changes regarding a new diagnosis. The perioperative nurse is required to teach many aspects of the care including preoperative and postoperative treatments and medications.

Specimens and Diagnostics

The Specimens and Diagnostics section (Figure 4-7) lists medical tests and procedures that are ordered by the physician. Each entry contains the test/procedure name, the date that the test/procedure should be performed, and whether or not the physician wants to be notified when the results are available.

	D	E	N
Tests/Procedures Results Reviewed By Physician			
Tests/Procedures CHEST X-RAY	AB		

Figure 4-7

Medical Charting Demystified

The nurse also documents if the test/procedure was performed and if the physician was notified according to the medical order. There are times when the test/procedure couldn't be performed as ordered such as if the patient ate within 12 hours of the test when no food should have been eaten. In this situation, the nurse documents the reason for cancelling the test/procedure in this section and follows up with a further explanation in the nurse's notes.

Safety and Activity

This section (Figure 4-8) is used to specify the patient's permitted activity level based on the physician's orders. Activity levels are typically described as:

- Bed rest
- Bathroom privilege
- Out of bed ad lib
- Out of bed with assistance
- Physical therapy

Each shift, the nurse documents whether or not the patient complied with the activity level and if not, further explanation is provided in the nurse's notes.

Also specified in this section is whether or not the institution's safety protocol was adhered to. These typically include:

- Two side rails are up
- Bed is in the lowest position
- Call bell within reach
- Falls precaution

	D	E	N
Activity Level: OOB	AB		
Safety: Call bell in reach	AB		
Number of Side Rails Up ___2___	AB		
Bed Position: Up Down	AB		
Call Bell Within Reach	AB		

Figure 4-8

	D	E	N
Discharge Needs Assessment:			
Home _____1/1/08___	AB		
Rehab Facility _____			
Subacute Facility _____			
Transfer _____			
Discharge	AB		
_____1/1/08_____			

Figure 4-9

Discharge Plan

The Discharge Plan section (Figure 4-9) contains a very brief summary of where the patient is going after leaving the unit based on a needs assessment. It does not contain the complete patient's discharge plan, which is usually provided in a different document.

Items in the Discharge Plan section are:

- Home
- Rehabilitation facility
- Subacute facility
- Transfer
- Discharge

Summary

With the nursing process as a foundation, the care plan is a road map that guides the healthcare team when caring for a patient. There are three basic components of any care plan: the patient's problems, interventions used to address each problem, and the expected outcome of those interventions.

Patient's identified problems are always described as a nursing diagnosis defined by NANDA. A goal is set for actions taken by the healthcare team to address each problem. An action is something done to achieve goals that were set for the patient. There must be a scientific basis for each action. Every action is evaluated to determine if the goal was reached. Goals are not always 100 percent achieved.

There are many formats used for a care plan and a care map. All serve as a guide for providing care to the patient. They differ in the format style and the kind of information contained in the care plan. Care plans are either student care plans or institutional care plans; an institutional care plan is usually part of the care map, which provides the comprehensive plan for the patient, making it an interdisciplinary tool of care.

Quiz

1. The nurse is evaluating the plan of care for a patient and determines that a problem still exists. The FIRST revision to the plan of care is:

   a. The problem

   b. The intervention

   c. The nursing diagnosis

   d. The goal

2. The nurse preparing a plan of care for a patient will formulate the plan based on the:

   a. Medical diagnosis

   b. Nursing diagnosis

   c. Nursing process

   d. Discharge needs

3. The nurse initiates an intervention that:

   a. Has a scientific rationale

   b. Has a measureable outcome

   c. Is specific to the patient

   d. All of the above

4. The nurse is caring for a patient with a nursing diagnosis of impaired skin integrity related to a stage 1 pressure ulcer. The most appropriate goal for this patient is:

   a. The patient will not get any more pressure ulcers.

   b. The patient's ulcer will decrease in size from 3 to 2 cm in 1 week.

   c. The patient's ulcer will start to heal.

   d. The patient's skin will not break down.

5. The nurse auscultates rales in the base of her patient's right lung field. Which part of the care map/care plan will the nurse reflect that information?

   a. Assessment

   b. Diagnosis

   c. Intervention

   d. Evaluation

6. When is the most appropriate time to create a care plan?

    a.   When the patient is transferred to the unit

    b.   At the request of the physician

    c.   At the request of the nurse supervisor

    d.   When the patient is admitted

7. When is the most appropriate time to modify a care plan?

    a.   Never

    b.   Upon readmission

    c.   Following assessment of the patient

    d.   At the request of the physician

8. Who can modify a care plan?

    a.   The admitting nurse

    b.   The primary nurse

    c.   The licensed practical nurse (LPN)

    d.   The patient

9. What is the goal of a care plan?

    a.   Provide a comprehensive plan for a patient's care

    b.   Provide a check list of tasks for the primary nurse

    c.   Provide a check list of tasks for the nursing staff

    d.   Give the physician guidance for caring for the patient

10. What type of care plan uses scientific rationale?

    a.   Student and institutional care plans

    b.   Institutional care plans

    c.   Student care plans

    d.   Scientific rationales are never included in a care plan

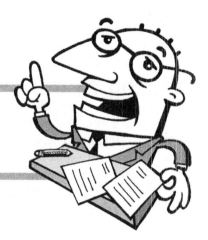

CHAPTER 5

Acute Care Charting

A chart is like a connect-the-dot puzzle where each dot is objective or subjective data about the patient reported by a member of the healthcare team. The patient's problem is identified by connecting these dots and then a plan is devised to care for the patient.

A critical aspect of the nurse's job is to translate results of your assessment of the patient into terms that accurately describes the patient's condition, which is similar to how a newspaper report finds the best words to describe a news event.

Sometimes you are provided with printed or electronic forms that contain a list of words used to describe common patient assessments. You simply pick the appropriate word from the list to describe your patient's assessment.

Other times, blank forms are used such as a patient's progress note where you need to come up with the proper words to describe your patient's assessment. Finding the best words can be challenging for the new nurse who isn't proficient at charting an assessment.

In this chapter, you'll learn the words of charting.

Writing in the Chart

You learn how to chart your assessment during your clinical rotations in nursing schools. The style of charting (see Chapter 1) depends greatly on the healthcare facility, nursing school, and clinical instructor.

Some clinical instructors might prefer new nursing students to chart both normal and exceptional findings of their patient's assessment. Advanced students are typically required to chart only exceptions of normal findings, which is the style of charting used in most healthcare facilities. You'll find that we've included words that describe both normal findings and exceptional findings that you may encounter during your assessment.

Abbreviations are frequently used when charting as a way to reduce the time and space needed to write your notes. Table 5-1 shows some abbreviations that are commonly used. Check your healthcare facility's list of approved and prohibited abbreviations as published by the Joint Commission on Accreditation of Healthcare Organizations (JCAHO) with regard to the patient safety goals.

Healthcare facilities and clinical instructors decide on how you will describe your patient's assessment in the chart. At times you may be asked to tell how you found the patient when you first entered the room. You might write:

Pt in bed, awake, A&O times 3, bed in low position, 2 SR↑, call bell in reach, daughter at bedside. ID band on.

This description is then followed by your head-to-toe assessment of the patient as shown in Figure 5-1. The remaining pages of this chapter contain words and phrases that you can use to describe your patient's condition.

Table 5-1   Abbreviations Used in Charting

Abbreviation	Description	Abbreviation	Description
PT	Patient	R in a circle	Right
SR	Side rails	LW	Left wrist
RM	Room	RW	Right wrist
Bilat	Bilateral	BR BRP	Bathroom Bathroom privilege
L in a circle	Left	BM	Bowel movement
OOB	Out of Bed	P	Pulse
Resp	Respiration	T	Temperature
BP	Blood pressure	Cap refill	Capillary refill
AC A&O CTA	Antecubital Alert and oriented Clear to auscultation	S with a line over C with a line over WNL	Without With Within normal limits

Progress Notes
19:00 PT in bed, low position. HOB 30 degrees. 2 SR_. Call bell in reach. ID ban on.
Bed rest. Wife at bedside. NPO. BP 161/90 T 98.3 Rep 26 P 80 bounding. POX 96 on rm
air. pain 2 (0–10), oriented X3, cooperative, PERL, smile symmetric, no deviation of
tongue, no productive cough, lungs R upper lung wheezing, R lower, L clear)
telemetry #29 NSR. IV sit .45 NS 100 mL/hr L wrist heparin lock, 20 gauge clear,
dry via pump. Cap refill <3 sec, Hand grip equal, bowel sounds X4 quad, void +
BM unassisted in bed pan. Pitting edema R Leg 1+ L Leg 1+. Equal pressure bilat
feet, Pedal Pulse strong bilat. Wound L Inferior calf laceration with sutures clean
dry intact. VAC dressing CDI to −125 mm Hg draining serosangunous drainage.

Figure 5-1

APPEARANCE

Normal

Posture (erect/relaxed)

Body movement (voluntary/deliberate/coordinated/smooth and even)

Dress (appropriate for setting, season, age, gender, social group/clothing fits)

Grooming and hygiene (hair is neat and clean/facial hair shaved or well groomed/nails clean)

Abnormal

Posture (curled in bed/darting watchful eyes/restless pacing/sitting slumped/dragging feet/slow walking/sitting at edge of bed)

Body movement (restless/fidgety/facial grimace/unsteady gait/uncoordinated)

Dress (inappropriate for setting, season, age, gender, social group/clothing does not fit)

Grooming and hygiene (unilateral neglect/poor hygiene/lack of concern about dress/ungroomed/disheveled)

BEHAVIOR

Normal

Level of consciousness (awake/alert/aware/oriented/recent memory/ judgment/mood/affect)

Facial expression (appropriate/changes with topic/eye contact)

Speech (effortlessly/clear/shares conversation/fluent/understandable/forms words/completes sentences/native language/articulation/pattern)

Mood and affect (appropriate/cooperative)

Abnormal

Level of consciousness (lethargic/obtunded/stupor/semicoma/coma/confused/disoriented)

Facial expression (flat/masklike/grimacing)

Mood and affect (flat)

Speech (dysphonia/monopolizes conversation/silent/secretive/uncommunicative/slow/monotonus/rapid-fire/pressures/loud/dysarthria/misuses words/omits words/transposes words/repetitious/long delay in finding word/failure in word search/nonverbal/garbled)

Mood and affect (flat/blunted/anxiety/fear/irritability/rage/ambivalence/lability/euphoria/elation/depersonalization/depression/dulled concentration/impaired judgment/uninhibited/talkativeness/impaired memory/irritability)

Pain (as per pain scale)

NUTRITION

Normal

Skin (smooth/no rashes/no bruises/flaking)

Hair (shiny/firm/healthy scalp)

Eyes (clear/shiny/membranes pink and moist/no sores at corners of eyelids)

Lips (smooth/not chapped/not swollen/pink/not cracked)

Tongue (red/not swollen/not smooth/no lesions)

Gums (reddish pink/firm/no swelling/no bleeding)

Nails (smooth/pink/clean)

Abnormal

Skin (dry/flaking/scaly/petechiae/ecchymoses/bumpy/cracks/lesion/hyperpigmentation/rash/bruise)

Hair (dull/dry/sparse/corkscrew hair/color changes/falls out easily)

Eyes (dryness/pale conjunctivae/red conjunctivae/softening/foamy plaques)

Lips (vertical cracks on lips/red cracks at sides of mouth)

Tongue (beefy red/pale/papillary atrophy/papillary hypertrophy/purplish)

Gums (bleeding)

Nails (brittle/ridged/spoon-shaped/splinter/hemorrhages/striata/jagged/bitten/dirty/clubbing/cyanotic/spongy/pits/transverse grooves/lines)

VITAL SIGNS

Normal

Pulse (write value)

Blood pressure (write value)

Pain (absent)

Abnormal

Pulse (full/bounding/weak/thready/absent)

Blood pressure (write abnormal value)

Pain (burning/stabbing/aching/throbbing/firelike/squeezing/cramping/sharp/itching/tingling/shooting/crushing/dull/crying/moaning/pain when palpated/clutching area)

SKIN

Normal

Color (freckle [ephelis]/mole [nevus]/junctional nevus/birthmark/diameter in millimeters/senile lentigines)

IV sites (clean, dry, intact with no signs of redness/no signs of infiltration)

Temperature (write temperature)

Moisture (warm/dry)

Texture (smooth/soft/no dryness/no cracking/no rashes)

Thickness (normal/uniform)

Edema (none)

Turgor (no tenting)

Abnormal

Color (brown/tan/black-blue [ecchymosis]/red (erythema)/white/yellow/ ashen gray/asymmetrical pigment/border notching/border scalloping/border ragged edges/border poorly defined margins/pencil eraser size/elevated/ keratosis)

Dressings (wound drainage [serosanguineous, purulent, sanguineous, scant/ saturated/red-brown])

IV sites (not clean, not dry, not intact/signs of redness/infiltration, cool, swollen/phlebitis, red, warm to touch)

Temperature (hyperthermia/hypothermia)

Moisture (diaphoresis/dry/parched/cracked)

Texture (velvetlike/rough/dry/flaky/blisters)

Thickness (very thin/shiny/atrophic/callus)

Edema (1+/ 2+/3+/4+ pitting)

Turgor (tenting)

LESIONS

Normal

Description (no lesions)

Abnormal

Description (annular/circular/begins in center/spreads/run together/ confluent/discrete/distinct/grouped/clustered/target/polycyclic/together/ zosteriform/linear arrangement/linear/scratch/streak/line/stripe/gyrate/ twisted/coiled/spiral/snakelike/flat/less than/greater than/solid/elevated/ hard/soft/deep/shallow/superficial/raised/transient/dried-out exudate/ honey-colored/weeping/shedding/silver/micalike/yellow/greasy/depressed/ smooth/rubbery/clawlike)

Type (macule/patch/nodule/wheal/fluid held/urticaria/hives/vesicle/bulla/ cyst/pustule/crust/scale/linear crack/abrupt edges/fissure/erosion/ulcer/ scar/lichenification/prolonged intense scratching/excoriation/atrophic scar/keloid/hypertrophic scar/port-wine stain/strawberry mark/spider/star/ purpura/petechiae/venous lake)

EYES

Normal

Eyes (iris intact/conjunctivae clear/sclerae white/cornea intact/ PERRLA [pupils equal round reactive to light and accommodation] perrla)

Abnormal

Eyes (lower lid dropping away/lower lid turning in/lids edematous/ discolored/swollen/almost shut/inward turn of eye/outward turn of eye/ inward drift/outward drift/periorbital edema/protruding eyes/drooping upper lid/light-colored areas in outer iris/large space between eyes/inflammation of eyelids/stye/inflammation of lacrimal sac/nodule protruding on lid/infective conjunctivae/circumcorneal redness/subconjunctival hemorrhage/corneal abrasion/unequal pupil/constricted pupils/fixed pupils/sluggish reaction to light/enlarged pupils/pupils no response to light)

EARS

Normal

Ears (no tenderness/no discharge/no masses/no lesions/canals clear of cerumen/able to hear whispered voice bilaterally)

Abnormal

Ears (reddish-blue discoloration of auricle/swelling/skin tag/painful movement of the pinna/purulent discharge/scaling/itching/clear fluid discharge/infected hair follicle)

NOSE, MOUTH, THROAT

Normal

Nose (naris patent/mucosa pink/nontender/no lesions/no obstruction/ mobile/no discharge/no swelling)

Mouth and throat (muscoa pink/no lesions/uvula midline/rises on phonation/tonsils present/no lumps/tonsils)

Abnormal

Nose (mucosa gray and boggy/tender/lesions/obstruction/not mobile/ discharge)

Mouth and throat (coated tongue/dry mouth/absent salivation/decreased salivation/increased salivation/lesions/plaque/pain/ulcers/vesicles/purulent drainage/hemorrhagic/edema/no tonsils/coughing/aspiration/regurgitation/ white cheesy curdlike patch/chalky white thick raised patches/borders well defined/blue-white spots/irregular red halo)

BREASTS

Normal

Location (upper inner quadrant/upper outer quadrant/lower inner quadrant/ lower outer quadrant/auxiliary tail of Spence)

Abnormal

Breasts (thickening/swelling/changes in bra size/rash/tenderness/ hyperpigmentation/dimpling/pucker)

Discharge (color/thick/runny/odor/first noticed)

Lump (location/width/length/thickness/oval/round/lobulated/indistinct/soft/ firm/hard/movable/fixed/single/multiple/erythematous/dimpled/retracted/ tender)

LUNGS

Normal

Location (anterior axillary line/midclavicular line/midsternal line/scapular line/vertebral line/posterior axillary line/midaxillary line/right upper lobe [RUL]/right middle lobe [RML])/right lower lobe [RLL]/left upper lobe [LUL]/left lower lobe [LLL])

Palpation (chest symmetrical/tactile fremitus equal bilaterally/no lumps/no tenderness)

Resonance (equal bilaterally)

Adventitious sounds (none/clear to auscultation/clear to all lung fields)

Abnormal

Cough (continuous/afternoon/evenings/night/early morning/streak blood/ frank blood/sputum production/color/amount/hacking/dry/barking/hoarse/ congested/bubbling/occurs on lying)

Respiration (shortness of breath/hard breathing/tachypnea/bradypenia/ hyperventilation/hypoventilation/Cheyne-Stokes)

Tactile fremitus (decrease/increase/rhonchi/pleural friction/crepitus/crackling)

Resonance (dull/hyperresonance)

Adventitious sounds (fine crackles/coarse crackles/rales/pleural friction rub/wheeze on inspiration and/or expiration/stridor/rhonchi/absent or decreased or diminished)

CARDIAC

Normal

Chest pain (none)

Skin (pink)

Carotid artery (no bruit/normal pulse/no distention)

Pain (no pain)

Abnormal

Chest pain (crushing/stabbing/burning/viselike/duration)

Pain brought on by (rest/emotional upset/after eating/during intercourse/ cold weather/pain at rest)

Pain worsened by (moving arm/moving neck/breathing/lying flat)

Associated symptoms (pale skin/skips beat/shortness of breath/nausea/ vomiting/fast rate/ number of pillows used to sleep)

Skin (ashen/pallor/cyanosis/cool, clammy/diaphoretic)

Carotid artery (bruit/diminished pulse/increase pulse/strong pulse/ distention/bounding)

PERIPHERAL VASCULAR

Normal

Skin (pink)

Visualized veins (none observed)

Cramp (one)

Abnormal

Cramp (burning/aching/cramping/stabbing/gradually/suddenly/awaken at night/worse in cool weather/worse when elevated/aching)

Cramp relieved by (dangling/walking/rubbing/stop walking)

Skin (red/pallor/blue/brown)

Visualized veins (bulging/crooked/ulcer/swollen/distended/torturous)

GASTROINTESTINAL

Normal

Food intolerance (none)

Stomach/abdominal pain (none)

Bowel (last BM/well formed/normal color/bowel sounds present X4)

Appetite (normal)

Weight (no change)

Abdominal contour (flat/rounded/obese)

Abdomen (no mass/no tenderness/soft/not tender/not distended)

Abnormal

Food intolerance (heartburn/belching/bloating/indigestion/allergic reaction)

Stomach/abdominal pain (moves around/aggravated by movement/dull/general/poorly localized/sharp/precisely localized/aggravating factors/alleviating factors/difficulty swallowing/bulging location/firm/rigid/distended/guarded)

Bowel (last BM/tarry stool/red stool/gray stool)

Appetite (loss appetite)

Weight (increase unexpected/decrease unexpected)

Abdominal contour (scalphoid/protuberant)

Abdomen (dull/distended/hyperresonance/pulsating/systolic bruit)

MUSCULOSKELETAL

Normal

Joint (no tenderness /no swelling/full ROM/no stiffness/no deformity/not tender)

Abnormal

Joint (redness/swelling/heat/tenderness/limited ROM/stiffness/tender/nodules/deformity)

Neurologic

Normal (also see Behavior)

Head/mental status (alert/oriented to person, place, time/cooperative/recent memory/judgment/mood/affect/speech clarity/articulation/pattern/content appropriate/native language/facial expression/PERRLA [pupils equal round reactive to light and accommodation])

Peripherals (dorsiflexion/plantar flexion/reflex)

Gait (tandem walking/smooth/rhythmic/effortless/coordinated)

Abnormal

Head (headache/dizziness/lightheaded/vertigo/feeling that you are spinning/feeling that room is spinning/syncope/aura/seizures/shaking/difficulty speaking/difficulty swallowing/uncoordinated/lethargic/obtunded/stupor/semicoma/delirium)

Peripherals (tremors/burning/tingling/numbness/muscle weakness)

Gait (stiff/unsteady/rigid arms/ataxia/staggering/crooked line of walk)

Summary

The nurse and other members of the patient's healthcare team observe, test, and ask a lot of questions to elicit data points that can be connected together to identify a patient's problem. Data points are recorded in the patient's chart.

These findings are both objective, such as the patient's blood pressure and pulse, and subjective, such as the color of the patient's skin. The healthcare team uses standard terms to describe objective and subjective findings.

Student nurses are frequently required to describe both normal and abnormal findings while healthcare institutions typically "chart by exception" where only abnormal findings are recorded in the patient's chart.

It is critical that the patient's healthcare team use abbreviations, words, and phrases that accurately communicate the findings to others on the team. Healthcare institutions typically specify abbreviations that can and cannot be used in a patient's chart. Medical terms have precise definitions; therefore the student nurse must be sure that the findings correspond exactly to a medical term before using the term to describe the patient's condition. Whenever you are in doubt, describe the findings in nonmedical term. Always remember that the goal is to accurately communicate the patient's condition to the healthcare team.

Quiz

1. Your patient is a 72-year-old man who is 12 hours' post open cholescystectomy. Your report from the previous nurse indicated the following: alert and oriented times 3, pleasant, cooperative, and appropriate, surgical dressing dry and intact, vital signs within normal limits, pain level 2/10 as per pain scale. When you evaluate the patient for your a.m. assessment, he calls you by his daughter's name, shows facial grimacing with incisional palpation, unable to describe pain level, and tells you that he's late for work. What would you write in his chart?

   a. Alert and oriented, denies pain, agree with previous assessment.

   b. Confusion to place

c. Alert, disoriented to place, responses inappropriate, demonstrates facial grimacing with incisional palpation, pain level indeterminable

   d. None of the above

2. The nurse is assessing the patient's wound dressing and visualizes a large, dark area of red blood on the dressing. The nurse makes a note in the chart describing this as:

   a. Purulent drainage

   b. Sanguineous drainage

   c. Scant serosanguineous drainage

   d. Dressing dry and intact

3. The nurse is assessing the patient's left lower ankle and notes edema. She presses on the patient's ankle and leaves a deep indentation. She includes in her note the following:

   a. 3+ pitting edema present to left ankle

   b. Some edema noted

   c. 1+ edema, no pitting

   d. Swollen ankle

4. The macule on the patient's left arm is described as a flat, uneven, light brown color spot.

   a. True

   b. False

5. The nurse is caring for a patient with orthostatic hypotension. The nurse's assessment concurs with that diagnosis. The most accurate documentation of that assessment is:

   a. Patient appears to be dizzy when standing.

   b. Patient complains of dizziness while ambulating.

   c. Patient's blood pressure lying down is 148/86; when patient stands at bedside blood pressure is 132/70.

   d. Morning assessment BP 150/92

6. The nurse is assessing lung sounds. Documentation for the assessment of abnormal breath sounds is best stated as:

   a. Lungs clear to ausculation

   b. Upper airway rhonchi heard to anterior chest, clear with coughing, bases clear bilaterally

c.   Rales heard

    d.   Rhonchi scattered

7. The nurse receives a report from the night shift that the patient's left peripheral IV site is clean and dry. When doing the a.m. assessment, the he notes that the IV site now appears cool to touch and swollen. The nurse's assessment is best stated as:

    a.   Left peripheral IV site swollen and cool to the touch. IV discontinued.

    b.   Phlebitis noted to left peripheral IV site.

    c.   IV site is clean and dry; no redness or swelling noted.

    d.   Infiltrated IV site.

8. Which note below best describes the patient's chest pain?

    a.   Patient complains of chest pain and states that it's really bad.

    b.   Patient points to chest and says the pain is unbearable.

    c.   Complaints of chest pain, 9/10 per pain scale, described by patient as "crushing."

    d.   Crushing pain to chest noted.

9. The nurse is caring for a postoperative patient with an abdominal incision. At 6 p.m., he gave the patient morphone sulfate (MS) 3 mg IVP for pain described as 9/10 per pain scale and at 6:30 he returned to reevaluate the pain level. The evaluation is best documented by stating:

    a.   Pain is better.

    b.   Pain has decreased from the rate 9/10 to rate 4/10.

    c.   Pain is 4/10.

    d.   Abdominal pain decreased from rate of 9/10 to rate 4/10 and described as "bearable"; resting quietly.

10. The day nurse charts for her end of shift note that the patient is lethargic. The night nurse expects to find the patient:

    a.   Fast asleep

    b.   Awake, alert, and oriented

    c.   Sleepy but arousable

    d.   Confused and disoriented

CHAPTER 6

Computer Charting

Paper charts are being replaced with computer charts in many healthcare facilities, resulting in a more efficient way to record and share patient information. However, computer charts are still vulnerable to many of the same errors as paper charts and can introduce new errors into a patient's record.

You probably can use a computer to surf the Internet, check your email, write a paper using Microsoft Word, and find your way around popular computer applications. And if you haven't, that's fine too because you don't have to become a computer whiz to chart patient information on a computer.

There are three tasks you need to do to become proficient in computer charting. Know which keys to press, know what happens to patient information after you press those keys, and practice charting patient information. We'll show what keys to press and what happens after you press them. You'll need to practice on your own using your healthcare facility's computer charting application.

In this chapter, we'll demystify computing by taking you behind the scenes of a typical healthcare facility's computing system. The remaining chapters show how to use computers for charting.

Parts of the Computer Charting System

The first thing that usually comes to mind when reading the term *computer charting* is a healthcare professional looking at a computer screen and keyboard. The computer screen is just one of many parts of a computer charting system. The other parts are hidden from sight because you don't need them to use the computer charting system.

There are six major parts of a computer charting system. These are:

1. Computer workstation
2. Network
3. Server
4. Database
5. Printers
6. Charting program

COMPUTER WORKSTATION

A computer workstation is a PC (personal computer) used to chart patient information. Some healthcare facilities have a PC at each nurse's station and others also have a laptop PC that can be moved to the patient's room. Although they are referred to as a computer workstation in the healthcare facility, these are the same PCs that you might have at home.

A PC or any computer for that matter is a box of switches (see Workstation: An Inside Look). A special group of computer programs called an operating system enables those switches to store and manipulate information. Arguably, the most widely used operating system is Microsoft Windows, which you probably use on your home computer. This is likely to be the operating system used on the workstation in your healthcare facility.

NETWORK

Workstations are connected together by a computer network (see Network: An Inside Look) called an intranet (Figure 6-1). Think of a network as a highway over which patient information travels. The network is a highway of cables that stretch from each workstation through the walls and floors and into a central room called a data center that contains other computers called servers (see Server) that consolidate patient information into a database (see Database).

Some workstations might be connected to the network through a wireless connection called a wifi where patient information is transmitted to a receiver that

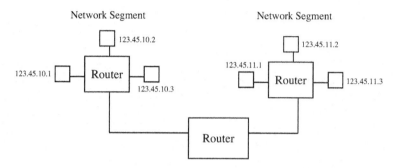

Figure 6-1   A computer network.

is connected to the network via a cable. This is the same way your favorite song is transmitted by a radio station to your radio. The only difference is that the wifi transmitter sends encrypted (see Encryption) patient information within the healthcare facility.

DATABASE

A database is a collection of data. You create a patient's database by gathering objective and subjective information about the patient through your assessment. With computerized charting, the database is an electronic collection of data from all patients.

Think of the database as an electronic filing cabinet containing patient information that can be stored and accessed using a workstation over the healthcare facility's computer network. This is very similar to how you access your bank account information from your home PC over the Internet.

PRINTERS

The trend is to replace printing information on paper with displaying the information on a computer screen. However, realistically you'll always need to print something, which is why you'll find a printer at the nurse's station.

A printer is connected to the network, enabling workstations to share the same printer. In addition, workstations can use other printers on the network by choosing a printer from a list of available printers (see Chapter 7) when you print. If the printer at your nurse's station isn't working, you can use the printer at the nearest nurse's station.

CHARTING PROGRAM

You probably have heard the term computer program if you have a home computer. There are many computer programs available, each of which lets you do something unique with your computer such as word processing using Microsoft Word.

A charting program lets you use the computer to record, retrieve, edit, and print a patient's chart. There are many different kinds of charting programs available, all of which are used to electronically chart patient information; however, each does so in a slightly different way. We'll show you how to use features found in many charting programs in the next chapter.

Workstation: An Inside Look

A workstation is similar to your computer and is used to enter, store, transmit, receive, and display information such as emails, web pages, and patient information. It has many features found on your computer, so you probably have an idea on how to use the workstation.

The keyboard and mouse are used to enter information into the charting program and other programs that your healthcare facility has on the workstation. However, you might notice other devices used to input data, such as, a bar code reader that is used in the supermarket.

A bar code reader scans bar codes that contain encoded information that is translated into data that that you can understand. Depending on the nature of the charting program, a bar code reader is used to scan employee IDs, patient's ID bracelets, bar codes on medication, laboratory specimens, and medical supplies. This saves time entering information into the workstation and increases the accuracy of the information by reducing the risk of typographical errors.

For example, before administering medication, the nurse scans her employee ID, scans the medication, and scans the patient's ID bracelet into the workstation. The workstation then verifies that the correct medication and dose is going to be administered to the right patient at the right time using the prescribed method of administration. A warning message is displayed if there is a discrepancy. If all the information is correct, the nurse then uses the keyboard or mouse to confirm that the medication was administered.

WHERE THE INFORMATION GOES

The information is temporarily stored in the workstation's memory and is sometimes also stored on the workstation's hard drive. Information stored in memory is erased automatically when the workstation is turned off. Information stored on the hard drive remains on the hard drive even after the workstation is off.

You don't have to worry about losing information because many charting programs automatically transmit information over the network to a data center rather than storing information on the workstation's hard drive. This is done for security reasons.

Furthermore, workstations are typically powered by circuits that are connected to the healthcare facility's back-up power supplies. Workstations remain operating during a power outage.

RETRIEVING AND DISPLAYING INFORMATION

In order to recall and display information, you'll be prompted to enter your ID and password that are provided to you by your healthcare facility. Your ID is granted rights to retrieve and display information that you are authorized to view based on HIPPA (Health Insurance Portability and Accountability Act) and the healthcare facility's policy. The healthcare facility's technology department assigns you those rights.

For example, after entering your ID and password (logging in), the charting program displays a list of patients assigned to you by the nurse manager. You are able to access information about those patients that you need to do your job. The charting program automatically hides information that you are not authorized to view.

Access to patient information might be limited. It is common for the workstation to automatically erase information from the screen and log you out after a period of time has passed to assure that the information remains secure. This reduces the risk that patient information can be viewed on the screen after you walk away from the workstation or that another person can use the workstation while you are still logged in.

DEMYSTIFIED DATA

If you are curious as to how words are stored inside your workstation, then be sure to read this section; otherwise skip it.

The workstation contains tiny electronic switches that can be turned on or off similar to a light switch. In order to store a character found on the keyboard to the workstation, the character must first be translated into a number that consists of a series of 0s and 1s called a binary number. This probably sounds too nerdy, but it is easy to understand.

There is a code book that assigns each keyboard character a binary number. When you press a key on the keyboard, a program inside the workstation looks up the letter in the code book and then reads the corresponding binary number.

Let's see how this works. Enter the word *nurse* into the workstation and these letters are translated in the binary numbers shown in Table 6-1.

The next step is storing these binary numbers into the electronic switches inside the workstation. Imagine for a moment that each switch is a light switch

Table 6-1   The Code Book

Keyboard Character	Binary Number
n	110 1110
u	111 0101
r	111 0010
s	111 0011
e	110 0101

that can be turned off and on. Let's say the off position is zero and the on position is one. Several light switches can be grouped together and its setting can be used to store a keyboard character.

Take a look at the first letter in Table 6-1. Each digit represents a light switch. The first two light switches are on, the third is off, the next three are on, and the last is off. By setting these switches accordingly, the letter "n" is stored inside the workstation.

The workstation displays keyboard characters by translating the switch settings (binary numbers) into images on the screen. The workstation screen is made up of tiny dots called pixels (picture elements). Think of these as tiny light bulbs. There are millions of them on a screen.

A program inside the workstation reads the setting of the light switches and then turns on the appropriate light bulbs on the screen to create the imagine of the corresponding keyboard character.

Network: An Inside Look

A computer network is a highway that connects together workstations, printers, and computing devices in the healthcare facility's data center. The network can also extend to physician offices, paramedic mobile units, medavac aircraft, and organizations that do business with the healthcare facility such as insurance companies, banks, and suppliers.

Any computing device (i.e., workstation) on the network can transmit data to another computing device by sending data over the network. For example, a physician can use the workstation at the nurse's station to send a medication order over the network to the pharmacy.

THE NETWORK IS YOUR HOMETOWN

You might wonder how this electronic highway works. It works like your hometown. Each workstation, printer, and other computing devices has a unique address called an IP address. Think of this as the address of your house. The street is the pathway to buildings in your town similar to how the network cable is the pathway to computing devices on the network.

When you want to send your friend who lives across town an invitation to a barbeque, you place the invitation in an envelope and write on the envelope your friend's address as the destination address and your address as the return address, and then give the envelope to the postal carrier who is driving down the street. The postal carrier delivers the envelope to your town's post office where the envelope is sorted and given to your friend's postal carrier who delivers it to your friend's house.

This is basically the same process that occurs when data are sent over a computer network. The envelope is an electronic envelope called a packet. The data that are to be sent are electronically placed into the packet and the packet is addressed with the destination computer's IP address and the IP address of the computer sending the packet. The packet is then sent along the network to a post office–like device called a router where the packet is then forwarded to the destination computer.

A computer network typically has several "towns," each referred to as a network segment (see Figure 6-1). Segments are connected to regional routers (regional post offices) via cable, enabling data to be easily transmitted to any network segment.

This is similar to how a county or parish is divided into many towns. Towns are connected together by county roads. And mail sent to a different town is first sent from the town's post office to a regional post office, where it is redirected to the other town's post office, which delivers the letter to its destination address.

HOW WORDS MOVE ALONG A CABLE

If you're curious as to how the electronic envelope travels across the network cable, then be sure to read this section; otherwise skip it.

Imagine for a moment a dishpan filled with water. The water is still. You can create a wave in the dishpan by moving a knife up and down in the water. Each time the knife is pushed down, water molecules are moved up, creating the wave. No wave is created when the knife is out of the water.

The 0s and 1s used to represent characters on the keyboard (see Demystifying Data) can be represented by a wave. The peak of the wave is 1 and no wave is 0. By pushing—and withholding—the knife in the water you could transmit a keyboard character across the dishpan.

Although this isn't very practical, it illustrates the concept used to transmit 0s and 1s over network cables. In networks, an electronic wave is created when electricity is applied to the cable. The electricity is controlled by circuits inside the computer that translates the 0s and 1s of the electronic envelope into the wave. Circuits in the destination computer translate electronic waves back to 0s and 1s and store them in switches inside the computer.

Transmitting Without Cable

You probably have noticed a customer or two using a laptop to surf the net at a table in an upscale coffee shop, or maybe you've done this yourself. The laptop didn't need a cable to connect to the Internet because the coffee shop provided a wifi connection—a wireless connection to the Internet.

Healthcare facilities are also using wifi technology to connect laptops to the healthcare facility's network. Laptops are mobile workstations that can be brought to each patient's room, enabling the nurse to update the patient's chart immediately after caring for the patient.

Wifi uses radio waves, which is the same technology used to broadcast radio programs only over a very short distance. Laptops and other mobile computing devices have a built-in wifi transceiver. This consists of circuits that can transmit a signal and receive a signal. Any receiver tuned to the wifi's frequency can receive the signal, but only authorized receivers can understand the data that are being transmitted.

All data are encrypted before being transmitted. Only a receiver with the proper cipher can decipher the data, and in this way protects the data from eavesdropping computer devices that connect to wifi.

Demystifying Wifi Transmission

Skip this section if you're not inquisitive about how data are transmitted through the air using wifi transmission.

Remember back to third grade science class when the teacher told you there are molecules of air all around you even though you cannot see or feel them. Air molecules are similar to water molecules that you used to move with the knife to create a wave in the dishpan (see How Words Move Along a Cable). You can push air molecules to create a wave.

Circuits in the wifi transceiver located inside a computing device sets air molecules in motion, creating a wave. Zeroes and ones are encoded by designating the peak of a wave as one and no wave or the bottom of the wave as zero.

Wifi technology replaces the cable in a network. Other network features such as the electronic envelop (packet) and IP addresses are used. The electronic envelop is transmitted over the wifi signal.

Database: An Inside Look

The patient's chart, patient billing, payroll, and employee information are just a few types of information that a healthcare facility must store and retrieve quickly in order to care for patients and pay their own bills. Most information is stored electronically, although some information must be stored in its original state as required by the healthcare facility's legal department.

Electronic information is stored in a database management system (DBMS). Think of this as an electronic filing cabinet and a super–file clerk all rolled up in one. The DBMS resides on a computer called a database server that is located in the healthcare facility's data center and is operated by a technician called a database administrator.

It is rare that you will directly use a DBMS. Instead, the DBMS interacts with other software such as the charting software that you use to care for your patients. For example, you'll select the patient's chart using the charting software and the charting software forwards your request to the DBMS. The DBMS searches its records for the information and sends the information over the network to the charting software, which then displays the information on the screen.

SECURITY ACCESS

HIPPA and other regulations in addition to good business practice require that access to a healthcare facility's computers and information stored in those computers be restricted on a need-to-know basis. Restrictions are enforced by setting security access for each employee to the healthcare facility's computers.

Each employee, who is permitted access to the healthcare facility's computers, is assigned a unique user ID and password. Behind the scenes, the user ID is permitted to access computer programs and information that corresponds to the security access settings assigned by the healthcare facility's information technology (IT) department.

User ID and Passwords

The IT department assigns you the user ID and creates a temporary password. You are prompted to change the password the first time you log into the computer. Only you know the password. The IT department cannot access your new password.

You must enter your user ID and password into the computer in order to use the charting program. These are validated by the computer against a known user ID and password.

A rejection message is displayed if there is a mismatch of user ID and password or if the user ID is inaccurate. You'll probably be given another opportunity to enter the correct user ID and password, depending on the healthcare facility's security access policy. At some point, the user ID will become suspended if it continues to be rejected. Typically, this occurs after three failed attempts.

The IT department can reinstate your user ID and password once it is satisfied you are who you say you are. The healthcare facility's policy dictates how you do this. For example, you might have to visit the IT department and show them your employee ID card. The IT department then resets your password to a temporary password. You'll then have to change the password the next time you log into the computer.

LOG IN FREQUENTLY

There is a tendency to log into the computer, enter some information into the charting program, and then walk away from the computer to perform other patient care. This is a security risk for the healthcare facility because anyone could step up and use the computer without having to log in.

To prevent this unauthorized access, the IT department usually automatically logs out a user ID after a specific time period has transpired such as every 10 minutes. The user ID isn't suspended. It can be used again to log back into the computer.

ENCRYPTION

Encryption is a process of converting information to a meaningless series of letters and numbers that can be stored or transmitted with little chance of anyone who doesn't have the cipher to be able to convert it back to readable information.

At the heart of the conversion process is a mathematical formula that uses a value called a key to transform meaningful information into meaningless information (encryption) and meaningless information to meaningful information (decipher).

Healthcare information is encrypted using a 128-bit key. The more bits in a key, the harder it is to break the encryption. A bit is a 0 or 1 (see Demystifying Data). You don't need to know any more about encryption because this is handled behind the scenes.

Hide Information in Plain Sight

Protecting patient information is challenging when the information is stored and accessed electronically. A major concern occurs when the information is displayed on the computer screen. Anyone walking in sight of the computer screen can view patient information displayed on the screen.

Healthcare facilities reduce the likelihood that the screen can be inappropriately viewed by automatically displaying a screen saver after a specified amount of time has passed. A screen saver is an image that is displayed when the computer is idle for a period of time. The healthcare facility's policy dictates the time period.

Another common technique used by healthcare facilities is to use a privacy filter over the screen. A privacy filter prevents anyone except the person in front of the computer from clearly seeing the image on the screen.

LIMITING CONTROL

Healthcare organizations whose stocks are traded publically must comply with the Sarbanes Oxley (SOX) Act. SOX was enacted in response to corporate scandals such as with Enron. SOX basically requires that checks and balance control must be implemented and enforced using computers. These are sometimes referred to as SOX controls. You probably won't experience SOX controls unless you work for a publically traded company.

A SOX control means that two or more persons should be responsible to complete a process to assure that one person does not have the capability to control a process from beginning to end. For example, a registered nurse (RN) can't reassign herself to another patient. This reassignment must be performed by the nurse manager.

PROTECTING ELECTRONIC INFORMATION

Patient information and other information needed for the healthcare facility to operate (i.e., billing information) are stored in databases in the healthcare facility's data center. The data center is especially designed to withstand many disasters such as power outages and fire.

Copies of databases and software such as the charting software are also stored off the premises in highly protected facilities usually operated by a vendor. These copies can be retrieved within hours should the on-site database becomes inaccessible.

In addition, some healthcare facilities have a duplicate contingency data center off premises that is immediately activated should the primary data center is unavailable.

A Tour of the IT Department

You'll probably have some encounter with your healthcare's IT department, whether it is to have your ID and password reset or serving on an advisory committee to help select a charting program. Therefore, it is probably a good idea to know how the IT department operates. The size and complexity of the IT department depends on the size of the healthcare facility. Larger facilities typically have more elaborate IT departments.

There are five groups found in most healthcare facility's IT departments. These are end user services, network, databases, applications, and administration.

The end user services group is responsible for the computer equipment on the unit and in the offices. You call them whenever anything goes wrong with your workstation or if new equipment needs to be ordered.

The network group is responsible for the hardware and software that is necessary to send and receive information over the computer network. Typically, they are called by the end user services group whenever there is a problem with the network. That is, you'll call the end user services group when your workstation isn't working properly. They call the network group if the trouble is with the network and not the workstation.

The database group is in charge of maintaining electronic information. It is their job to make sure that your patient's information is securely stored and available to the patient's healthcare team at a keystroke.

The applications group is in control of specialty programs such as the charting program that run on all computers in the healthcare facility. They are the in-house experts who you can call for assistance using that program.

The administration group sets the IT strategies and policies for the healthcare facility and oversees the operation of the other four groups within the IT division.

OUTSIDE HELP

Healthcare facilities frequently employ the services of outside IT experts to supplement their in-house staff. These are referred to as outsourced services because they involve IT tasks that are handled by a vendor rather than by the healthcare facility's employees.

Some healthcare facilities find outsourcing an economical way to provide IT services. For example, it might be less expensive to call in a repair technician to fix a workstation than to have the technician on staff because workstations don't frequently malfunction.

The degree in which IT services are outsourced greatly depends on the size of the healthcare facility. Small healthcare facilities are unable to afford a broad-skilled IT staff, and therefore find it financially sound to outsource most of IT services. In contrast, larger healthcare facilities have a greater demand for these services and find it economical to have an in-house staff.

Summary

A computer charting system stores and retrieves patient information using computer workstations, a network, and database. This information travels to and from workstations and databases over a network of cables and radio transmitters.

The workstation is nearly identical to a home PC. You use it the same way as you use your home computer. The network is similar to a private Internet called an intranet used to connect together computers within the healthcare facility. Think of the network as your hometown where computers are like houses, network cables are like streets, and the hub that keeps traffic flowing over the network is like the post office. Each computer is assigned a unique IP address, which is like your house address.

Information is placed in an electronic envelop called a packet. The packet is addressed with the destination IP address and the return IP address and then the packet is placed on the network where it is taken to an electronic post office (the router) and redirected to the destination computer.

Healthcare information that is stored and transmitted over the network must be encrypted using a 128-bit key. This makes it extremely difficult for anyone without the cipher to decode the information.

Computers, networks, and databases are controlled by the healthcare facility's IT department. The typical IT department has five groups: end user services, network, databases, applications, and administration.

Quiz

1. What is the major benefit of outsourcing IT tasks?

    a. It is a way to lower IT cost.

    b. It is a way to hire qualified IT technicians.

    c. It is a way to lower IT services.

    d. None of the above.

2. Why is a security filter placed on a computer display?

    a. Only to filter patient information from view.

    b. To decrease eye strain.

    c. To prevent viewing from straight in front of the display.

    d. To only allow viewing from straight in front of the display.

3. The best way to envision a computer network is as

    a. A cable

    b. A complex series of wires

    c. As your hometown

    d. As wifi

4. Patient information entered into charting software is stored in a database.

    a. True

    b. False

5. The best way to think of a DMBS is as an electronic filing cabinet and super–file clerk.

   a. True

   b. False

6. Encryption is

   a. Converting information into meaningless information using a key and mathematical formula

   b. Used to validate your user ID when logging into the computer

   c. Used by the network administrator to reject invalid log user IDs

   d. All of the above

7. You are automatically logged out of the computer as a security measure.

   a. True

   b. False

8. Wifi transmission of patient information can be intercepted.

   a. Yes, but the transmission is limited to the walls of the healthcare facility.

   b. Yes, but patient information is encrypted.

   c. No, because wifi is transmitted using a confidential frequency.

   d. None of the above.

9. Once logged into the computer, anyone using the computer has the same access as is granted to the user ID that is logged in.

   a. True

   b. False

10. Patient information is stored electronically in only one place.

   a. True

   b. False

CHAPTER 7

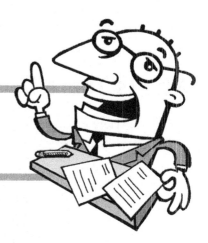

Charting Software

You use software every time you surf the Internet or when you email or text message your friends. There are all kinds of software programs, each tailoring your computer into a tool to perform a specific job such as playing music or showing pictures.

Charting software is similar to the software you use on your computer. It transforms the computer into a tool to document your patient's health electronically and shares patient information with the healthcare team no matter where they are located.

- No more paper and clumsy loose-leaf binder
- No more scratchy handwriting to decipher
- No more, "who has the chart?"

In this chapter, you'll learn your way around typical charting software, enough so that you can easily adapt what you learn here to any charting software used by your healthcare facility.

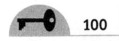

Why Is There Different Charting Software?

Here's a brief test:

What word processor do you use?

What spreadsheet do you use?

What operating system do you use?

Without thinking too long, you probably said Word, Excel, and Windows. There are other word processors, spreadsheets, and operating systems, but these are the most popular.

If you asked healthcare facilities what charting software they use, the response might surprise you because there isn't just one program used by every healthcare facility. Each facility chooses charting software from among several manufacturers who are prominent in the field.

DIFFERENT BUT SIMILAR

Although the healthcare industry uses different types of charting software, each works basically the same way. Regardless of who manufactured the charting software, you'll be able to:

- Select a patient from a list of your patients.
- Display the patient's electronic chart including the MAR (medication administration record), labs, and medical orders.
- Update the chart with your assessment of the patient.
- Enter orders.
- Order labs.
- And much more.

You will know how to use charting software even without reading this chapter because charting software has push buttons, drop-down lists, scrolling lists, text boxes, and other objects that you use in Microsoft Word, Excel, Windows, and other software.

Intuitively you'll know to double click a patient's name that appears in a list of patients if you want to see that patient's chart because you've selected information from a list in other software such as a document to open in Word. And you'll probably figure out that clicking a push button labeled Find starts a search for your patients.

Charting software differs from manufacturer to manufacturer in the way the chart is organized and the way information is entered and displayed. Think of this as similar to Microsoft Windows NT and Vista. Both do the same thing except differently, and Vista has more bells and whistles than Windows NT.

The best way to learn to use any charting software is to first find out how the charting software is organized and how to use its features.

Jumping In

The folks at McKesson, a leading manufacturer of charting software, agreed to let us walk you through how to use their software as a way to get your feet wet learning electronic charting. This chapter shows you how McKesson's software is organized and various ways to find your patient's chart. The remaining chapters show you how to enter your assessment of the patient, enter orders, review the MAR, and document other common tasks.

LOGGING IN

No doubt you've logged into a computer at school or work. A similar process is used to log into the healthcare facility's computer. You'll notice a login screen prompting you to enter your ID and password, which is assigned to each member of the healthcare team by the IT department.

Your ID is granted rights to access the healthcare facility's computerized charting software. Think of a right as a permission. This means anyone using your ID has the same rights because the computer thinks you are logged in. Therefore it is important not to share your ID and password with anyone.

Depending on your responsibilities and the policies of the healthcare facility, you are granted rights to various features of the software.

With charting software you might be granted rights to:

- Access the chart of some or all patients.
- Update some or all components of the chart.
- Delete information from chart.
- Reassign patients.
- Entering orders or specific types of orders.
- Accessing reports.

You might see different features on the screen than your supervisor sees because each of you has rights to different features of the software. For example, you may see a list of only your patients while your supervisor sees a list of all patients in the unit.

The Secret Password

The first time you log in you'll be asked to change your password. You can pick your own password. However, some healthcare facilities set minimum requirements for a password such as its length, and the combination of characters, numbers, and punctuation. You alone know your password.

You might also be asked to provide a question and answer to be used if you forgot your password. The question might be what school you attended. The answer is the name of your school. If you forget your password, you can click the reminder button on the login screen. The question is displayed and you're prompted to enter the answer. If correct, your password is emailed to you.

Your healthcare facility may require you to contact the IT department if you don't remember your password rather than let you click a password reminder button on the login screen. The IT department then resets your password and emails it to you. You'll be required to change the password the next time you log in. The IT department is not privy to your new password.

Frequent Logins

Expect to be required to log in frequently. Healthcare facilities have a policy requiring you to be automatically logged out if the computer sits idle for a few minutes. The assumption is that you walked away from the computer without logging off——and probably left your patient's information displayed on the screen.

The amount of time that needs to expire prior to being logged out is determined by the IT department. You can easily regain access by entering your ID and password into the login screen.

HINT *Moving the mouse every so often when you are spending a long time reading the screen can prevent you from being logged out.*

The Log

Your activities on the computer are probably recorded in an electronic log. An entry is made when you log in and when you log out. Entries might contain what software you use; what features of the software are used and what charts you viewed or changed. Nearly everything you do might be tracked.

Each log entry contains your ID; date and time that you gained access; the date and time that you terminated access; the unique ID of the computer you used; and other specific information about your activities.

The IT department refers to these entries whenever there is suspicion that the healthcare policy was violated. From time to time the healthcare facility and regulatory agencies may audit the log to assure compliance with policies and regulation.

HINT *Assume that everything you do using the healthcare facility's computers is being monitored including when you surf the Internet.*

IN THE BEGINNING

Charting software is used to store general information about the patient such as name, address, and insurance carrier and the patient's medical information.

The patient's chart begins when the admissions staff enters the patient's general information when the patient is admitted to the healthcare facility. This information is stored in a central database. Each member of the healthcare team electronically retrieves, at the click of the mouse, and updates the patient's chart to reflect their assessment and treatment plan.

If the patient was previously admitted to the healthcare facility, then the patient's information already exist in the database. The admissions staff and the patient's healthcare team then retrieve and update the information based on the patient's current condition.

LOCATING YOUR PATIENT'S CHART

There are a number of ways to find your patient's chart using charting software, the easiest of which is to select your patient from a list. Charting software displays a list of patients who are admitted to your unit called a census.

The list appears in a table (Figure 7-1) similar in appearance to a spreadsheet where each row represents a patient and columns contain key information about the patient such as:

	Notify	Last	First	Dept.	Rm/Bed	Diagnosis		Gen...	MRN	
0		DANIELS	MELANIE	24N	2400-1	(W) ABDOMINAL PAIN UNSPEC..		F	000001055	
1		EDGAR	MARNIE	24N	2400-2	(W) LUMP OR MASS IN BREAS..		F	000001054	
2		FREMONT	LISA CAROL	24N	2401-1	(W) PATHOLOGIC FX/UNSPEC..		F	000001060	
3		CRANE	LILA	24N	2402-1	(W) OTALGIA NOS (388.70)		F	000001056	
4		TYLER	BLANCHE	24N	2402-2	(W) NEUROTIC DEPRESSION (..		F	000001065	
5		DEVEREAUX	ANDRE	24N	2403-1	(W) CHEST PAIN NOS (786.50)		M	000001052	
6		BLANEY	RICHARD	24N	2403-2	(W) FEVER (780.6)		M	000001051	
7		LUMLEY	GEORGE	24N	2404-1	(W) CHEST PAIN NOS (786.50)		M	000001050	
8		OACKLEY	CHARLIE	24N	2406-1	(W) GASTROINTEST HEMORR..		M	000001061	
9		JEFFRIES	JEFF LB	24N	2407-2	(W) FLU W RESP MANIFEST N..		M	000001059	

Figure 7-1

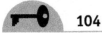

Notify	Last	/	First	Dept.	Rm/Bed	Diagnosis	Q	Gen..	MRN	▲
0	ARMSTRONG		MICHAEL	24N	2410-1	(W) CHEST PAIN NOS (786.50)	Q	M	000001053	
1	BLANEY		RICHARD	24N	2403-2	(W) FEVER (780.6)	Q	M	000001051	
2	CHILDRESS		ROBERT	24N	2408-1	(W) BRONCHITIS NOS (490), (F..	Q	M	000001149	
3	CRANE		LILA	24N	2402-1	(W) OTALGIA NOS (388.70)	Q	F	000001056	
4	DANIELS		MELANIE	24N	2400-1	(W) ABDOMINAL PAIN UNSPEC..	Q	F	000001055	
5	DEVEREAUX		ANDRE	24N	2403-1	(W) CHEST PAIN NOS (786.50)	Q	M	000001052	
6	EDGAR		MARNIE	24N	2400-2	(W) LUMP OR MASS IN BREAS..	Q	F	000001054	
7	EVERGUARD		ELIZABETH	24N	2409-1	(W) TACHYCARDIA NOS (785.0)	Q	F	000001121	▼
8	FREMONT		LISA CAROL	24N	2401-1	(W) PATHOLOGIC FX,UNSPEC..	Q	F	000001060	⊼
9	JEFFRIES		JEFF LB	24N	2407-2	(W) FLU W RESP MANIFEST N..	Q	M	000001059	⊻

Figure 7-2

- Notify
- Last Name
- First Name
- Department
- Room/Bed
- Diagnosis
- Gender
- Medical Record Number

Patients are sorted by information in one or more columns. The charting software determines the default sort order, which in McKesson's case is by room and bed. You can easily resort the list by clicking the column name that you want sorted. For example, clicking the Last Name column sorts the list by the patient's last name (Figure 7-2).

HINT *Notice that the list has the same scroll bar that you find on other Windows software. Click the up and down arrows to scroll incrementally. Drag the scroll bar to move quickly through the list. Click the top and bottom icons (below the down arrow) to jump to the top and bottom of the list.*

Filtering the List

Having the full list of patients at your fingertips comes in handy when you're covering a patient for another member of the healthcare team. Simply double click the patient's name and the charting software displays the patient's chart on the screen

However, you'll probably want to see some, but not all, patients' names based on whatever task that you are performing. You can do this by filtering the list to only patients that you need to see.

	Notify	Last	First	Dept.	Rm/Bed	Diagnosis		Gen..	MRN	
0		DANIELS	MELANIE	24N	2400-1	(W) ABDOMINAL PAIN UNSPEC..		F	000001055	
1		EDGAR	MARNIE	24N	2400-2	(W) LUMP OR MASS IN BREAS..		F	000001054	
2		FREMONT	LISA CAROL	24N	2401-1	(W) PATHOLOGIC FX,UNSPEC..		F	000001060	
3		CRANE	LILA	24N	2402-1	(W) OTALGIA NOS (388.70)		F	000001056	
4		TYLER	BLANCHE	24N	2402-2	(W) NEUROTIC DEPRESSION (..		F	000001065	
5		DEVEREAUX	ANDRE	24N	2403-1	(W) CHEST PAIN NOS (786.50)		M	000001052	
6		BLANEY	RICHARD	24N	2403-2	(W) FEVER (780.6)		M	000001051	
7		LUMLEY	GEORGE	24N	2404-1	(W) CHEST PAIN NOS (786.50)		M	000001050	
8		OACKLEY	CHARLIE	24N	2406-1	(W) GASTROINTEST HEMORR..		M	000001061	
9		JEFFRIES	JEFF LB	24N	2407-2	(W) FLU W RESP MANIFEST N..		M	000001059	

Figure 7-3

Above the table is a row of empty boxes; one for each column. Enter a value in the box and the charting software displays patients that have that value. Suppose you are assigned to department 24N and you want to see a list of patients who are admitted to that department. Enter the 24N in the empty box above the Dept. column and only those patients in department 24N are displayed on the screen (Figure 7-3).

HINT *Some empty boxes have drop-down lists such as department and gender have a drop- down list that contain valid values. You can pick a value only from the list provided in the drop-down list. You cannot enter a value that is not on the list. Other empty boxes such as last name and first name can accept any value.*

More Filtering

Whether you're viewing a list of all the patients or just your patients, you can use predefined filters to reduce the list to a specific category of patient. The categories can differ depending on the charting software; some charting software programs enable the healthcare facility to create their own categories.

For example, McKesson's charting software has three categories: type, status, and facility. Type describes if the patient is an inpatient, emergency, outpatient, in & out patient, or OB. Status is defined as active, discharged, pre-admit, and expired. And the facilities category identifies the division of the healthcare that is caring for the patient such as Link 3 East (the east wing of the third floor in the Link Building).

Categories are selected by picking the category from a drop-down box located at the bottom of the list. Click the Type down arrow to display the drop-down list and then click Inpatient to display a list of all inpatients (Figure 7-4).

Notify	Last	First	Dept.	Rm/Bed	Diagnosis	Gen..	MRN
0	DANIELS	MELANIE	24N	2400-1	(W) ABDOMINAL PAIN UNSPEC..	F	000001055
1	CHILDRESS	ROBERT	24N	2408-1	(W) BRONCHITIS NOS (490), (F..	M	000001149
2	ARMSTRONG	MICHAEL	24N	2410-1	(W) CHEST PAIN NOS (786.50)	M	000001053
3	DEVEREAUX	ANDRE	24N	2403-1	(W) CHEST PAIN NOS (786.50)	M	000001052
4	LUMLEY	GEORGE	24N	2404-1	(W) CHEST PAIN NOS (786.50)	M	000001050
5	MCKENNA	BEN	24N	2408-2	(W) CHEST PAIN NOS (786.50)	M	000001058
6	PICARD	MICHELE	24N	2411-1	(W) CHEST PAIN NOS (786.50)	F	000001064
7	BLANEY	RICHARD	24N	2403-2	(W) FEVER (780.6)	M	000001051
8	JEFFRIES	JEFF LB	24N	2407-2	(W) FLU W RESP MANIFEST N..	M	000001059
9	OACKLEY	CHARLIE	24N	2406-1	(W) GASTROINTEST HEMORR..	M	000001061

Type: All   **Status:** Active   **Facility:** Facility A

Census   Emergency   Outpatient   In & Out Pt   OB   All   lationship

Figure 7-4

Find Your Patients

Typically, you'll want to see only patients assigned to you for your shift by the nurse in charge. The McKesson's charting software does this when you click the Relationship tab (Figure 7-5).

Other charting software programs have a comparable feature. The relationship is both primary and secondary (covering) responsibility for the patient as determined by the nurse in charge. The charting software removes from the list all except your patients.

You might wonder how the charting software knows which patients are assigned to you. Staffing assignments are made using a management feature of the software that lists all patients in the unit and enables the nurse manager to assign each to a nurse and other members of the healthcare team.

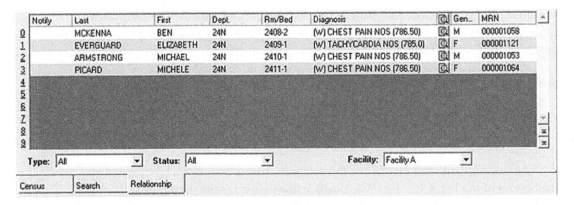

Notify	Last	First	Dept.	Rm/Bed	Diagnosis	Gen..	MRN
0	MCKENNA	BEN	24N	2408-2	(W) CHEST PAIN NOS (786.50)	M	000001058
1	EVERGUARD	ELIZABETH	24N	2409-1	(W) TACHYCARDIA NOS (785.0)	F	000001121
2	ARMSTRONG	MICHAEL	24N	2410-1	(W) CHEST PAIN NOS (786.50)	M	000001053
3	PICARD	MICHELE	24N	2411-1	(W) CHEST PAIN NOS (786.50)	F	000001064
4							
5							
6							
7							
8							
9							

Type: All   **Status:** All   **Facility:** Facility A

Census   Search   Relationship

Figure 7-5

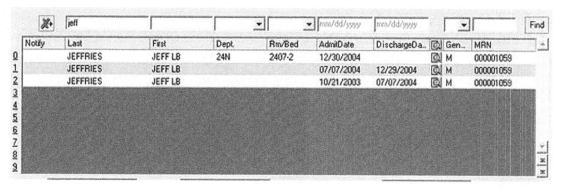

Figure 7-6

Partial Matches

In the real world, you may not know the correct spelling of a patient's name. However, this doesn't prevent you from locating the patient on the list. Enter a few letters of the patient's name, click the Find button, and let the charting software find patients that match.

Say that the patient's last name begins with Jeff. Enter these letters in the empty box over the Last Name column and McKesson's charting software displays possible matches (Figure 7-6) on the list. Of course, you'll still need to verify the patient.

In this example, McKesson's charting software displays all charts for the patient. Notice that the first row is missing a discharge date because the patient is currently admitted to the unit. Subsequent rows have the discharge date and are used to display the patient's charts from previous admissions.

DISPLAYING YOUR PATIENT'S CHART

Once you locate your patient on the list, the next step is to open the patient's chart on the screen by selecting the patient. Double click the row containing the patient's name and the charting software presents the patient's chart.

Figure 7-7 is the McKesson's chart for Elisabeth Everguard. At the top of the chart above the patient's name is a menu of features used to help analyze and manage information about this patient.

Below the menu contains information about the patient that you need at a glance. This includes the patient's account number and medical record number along with the patient's primary diagnosis.

Tabs divide the chart into sections similar to tabs in a ring binder chart. Clicking the tab opens the corresponding section of the charter where you can review and update the patient's information.

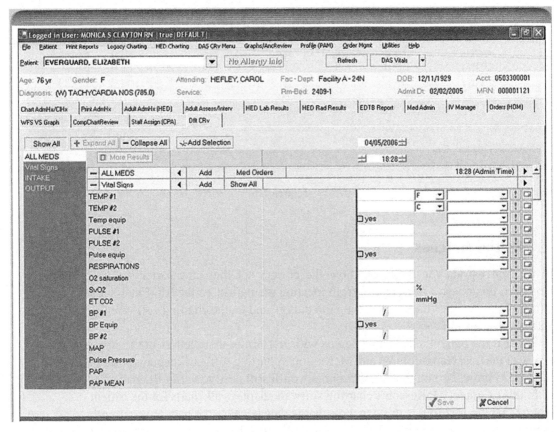

Figure 7-7

By default the chart is opened to the vital signs tab where you can quickly review the patient's status. You'll see how to enter vital signs and other patient information in the remaining chapters.

Summary

Charting software is similar to software that you use on your home computer. You use push buttons, drop-down lists, scrolling lists, text boxes, and other objects that you use in World, Excel, and other Windows software to interact with charting software.

Before you can access charting software, you must log into the healthcare facility's computers using your ID and password provided by the IT department. Your ID is granted rights to use some or all features in the charting software depending on your responsibility on the unit.

Your patient's electronic chart is created when the patient is admitted to the healthcare facility and is updated by the patient's healthcare team after the healthcare team assesses and treats the patient.

There are a number of ways to locate the patient using the charting software. You can scroll a list of patients or use the search feature of the charting software to find your patient. Once found, double clicking the patient's name displays the patient's chart.

Quiz

1. A computerized chart can be
   a. Reviewed simultaneously by different members of the healthcare team on different computers
   b. Restricted according to rights set by the IT department according to the healthcare facility's policies
   c. Be accessed by the patient's primary nurse
   d. All of the above

2. A patient's chart can be retrieved by the patient's Medical Record Number
   a. True
   b. False

3. The patient's nurse
   a. Can display the patient's previous charts from prior admissions
   b. Must print a copy of each section of the computerized chart after making changes to the chart
   c. Must print a copy of each section of the computerized chart before making changes to the chart
   d. Must provide the nurse manager with a printed copy of the computerized chart at the end of every shift

4. The nurse can display a list of the nurse's patients by diagnoses.
   a. True
   b. False

5. You interact with most charting software in the same way as you interact with programs on your home computer.
   a. True
   b. False

6. If the nurse is unsure of the correct spelling of the patient's name, the nurse
   a. Cannot use charting software to retrieve the patient's chart
   b. Can find the patient's chart by using a partial match search
   c. Must use the patient's ring binder chart
   d. None of the above

7. Most computer charts are divided into sections similar to sections found in a ring binder chart.
   a. True
   b. False

8. A computerized chart
   a. Can only be accessed by the patient's primary physician
   b. Cannot be accessed using a mobile computer on the unit
   c. Is stored in a central database
   d. None of the above.

9. The healthcare facility's computers automatically remove the computerized chart from the screen if there has been no interaction with the chart for a few minutes.
   a. True
   b. False

10. A member of the healthcare team who is not caring for a patient cannot access the patient's computerized chart.
    a. True
    b. False

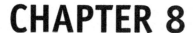

CHAPTER 8

To-Do List, Vital Signs, and I&O Charting

The days of taking the patient's ring binder chart to the bedside or trying to remember the patient's vital signs and I&O (input and output) until you get back to the nurses' station to record your findings are over. With the era of computerized charting, you can wheel a mobile computer running charting software directly to the patient's bedside.

Within a few mouse clicks you can quickly and efficiently record your patient's vital signs and fluids in charting software and then move on to your next patient. And your patient's information is made available to your patient's entire healthcare team immediately.

In this chapter, you'll learn how to record vital signs and I&O using charting software.

To-Do List

After getting a report during a shift change, the primary nurse needs to know what activities are scheduled for each patient in addition to routine vital signs and I&O. Charting software displays a To-Do List of activities that must be performed for the patient (Figure 8-1). Activities include scheduled medication, assessment, and labs.

Each patient is identified on a row on the To-Do List by the patient's name, unit, room/bed number, and medical record number. The entry also contains the name of an activity called Ordered Item and physician's order number. This enables you to quickly trace the activity back to the original physician's order.

In addition, you'll find information you need to perform the activity. For example, the activity might be to administer Fluorouracil Dextrose 5 percent to your patient. The entry in the To-Do List contains the dose, duration, route, and frequency. Furthermore, the entry indicates if the order is STAT (to be done immediately).

Each entry contains the date and time when the activity is scheduled. The Status column indicates whether the activity is overdue or not. You can also use a filter to see all activities that are overdue and you can also use a filter to see one patient or only your patients.

Patient Name	Scheduled	Group	Status	Ordered Item	Dose/Duration	Route	Prty Freq (Rate)	Order #'s	Comm
CRANE, LILA	05/22 10:00	IVS	Scheduled	FLUOROURACIL/DEXTROSE 5%	489 MG/1000 ML	IV	42 ml/hr	7544 (1)	CYTO
24N 2402-1 MRN:00000105	05/22 10:40	NSG	Overdue	ASSESS FOR CHEST PAIN	1 Occurrence		TODAY ONCE	2323858	
	05/22 10:50	LAB	Overdue	COMPLETE BLOOD COUNT	1 Occurrence		STAT STAT	2323866	
	06/22 17:00	LAB	Scheduled	COMPLETE BLOOD COUNT	1 Occurrence		ROUTINE ONCE	2323862	
TYLER, BLANCHE	05/22 12:00	DTY	Overdue	LOW TRIGLYCERIDE			DTY TIMED MEALS	2323667	
24N 2402-2 MRN:00000106	05/22 17:00	DTY	Scheduled	LOW TRIGLYCERIDE			DTY TIMED MEALS	2323668	
DEVEREAUX, ANDRE	05/22 10:39	NSG	Overdue	ASSESS FOR CHEST PAIN	1 Occurrence		TODAY ONCE	2323818	
24N 2403-1 MRN:00000105	05/22 17:00	LAB	Scheduled	COMPLETE BLOOD COUNT	1 Occurrence		ROUTINE ONCE	2323823	
JEFFRIES, JEFF LB	05/22 10:40	LAB	Overdue	COMPLETE BLOOD COUNT	1 Occurrence		TODAY ONCE	2323813	
24N 2407-1 MRN:00000105		NSG	Overdue	ASSESS FOR CHEST PAIN	1 Occurrence		TODAY ONCE	2323811	
CHILDRESS, ROBERT	05/22 10:00	IVS	Scheduled	POTASSIUM PHOSPHATE DIBASIC/D5W	5 MMOLE/1000 ML	IV	100 ml/hr	7651 (2)	
24N 2408-1 MRN:00000114	05/22 10:38	NSG	Overdue	ASSESS FOR CHEST PAIN	1 Occurrence		ROUTINE ONCE	2323804	
	05/22 17:00	LAB	Scheduled	COMPLETE BLOOD COUNT	1 Occurrence		ROUTINE ONCE	2323809	
EVERGUARD, ELIZABETH	05/22 10:41	NSG	Overdue	ASSESS FOR CHEST PAIN	1 Occurrence		TODAY ONCE	2323832	
24N 2409-1 MRN:00000112	05/22 12:00	DTY	Overdue	CARDIAC DIET			DTY TIMED MEALS	2323670	
	05/22 17:00	DTY	Scheduled	CARDIAC DIET			DTY TIMED MEALS	2323671	
		LAB	Scheduled	COMPLETE BLOOD COUNT	1 Occurrence		ROUTINE ONCE	2323837	
KENDALL, EVE	05/22 10:40	NSG	Overdue	ASSESS FOR CHEST PAIN	1 Occurrence		ROUTINE ONCE	2323825	
24N 2413-2 MRN:00000106	05/22 17:00	LAB	Scheduled	CBC (Complete Blood Count)	1 Occurrence		ROUTINE ONCE	2323830	
NEWTON, CHARLIE	05/22 10:40	NSG	Overdue	ASSESS FOR CHEST PAIN	1 Occurrence		ROUTINE ONCE	2323839	
24N 2414-2 MRN:00000106	05/22 17:00	LAB	Scheduled	COMPLETE BLOOD COUNT	1 Occurrence		ROUTINE Q12H	2323844	

Figure 8-1

Vital Signs

In Chapter 8, you learned how to display your patient's chart. The computerized chart is divided into sections similar to sections of the patient's ring binder chart. Each section is identified by a tab at the top of the computerized chart. Labels on tabs are usually determined by your healthcare facility.

The vital signs section of the McKesson's charting software is organized into groups called classes that appear in the left column and are referred to as the navigation panel. The classifications are ALL MEDS, VITAL SIGNS, I&O SUMMARY, INTAKE, and OUTPUT. Double clicking a classification with the mouse opens the classification in either Review Mode or Chart Mode, which lets you enter new vital signs into the chart.

Review Mode displays previous entries such as vital signs shown in Figure 8-2. You can use the right scroll bar to scroll down and up the list of vital signs and use the horizontal scroll bar at the bottom of the screen to scroll right or left to see a history of the patient's vital signs.

ENTERING VITAL SIGNS

Click the Chart button (see Figure 8-2) to enter the Chart Mode so you can enter new vital signs for the patient. The charting software automatically enters the date

	05/22/2006 10:12	05/22/2006 10:15	05/22/2006 11:37	05/22/2006 12:23	05/22/2006 12:51
Vital Signs — Chart					
TEMP #1		101.3F	103F Oral	103.5F Oral	
TEMP #2					
Temp equip		Yes			
PULSE #1		72			
PULSE #2					
RESPIRATIONS		22			
O2 saturation					
ET CO2					
BP #1		88/155		146/98	
BP Equip					
BP #2					
MAP					
Pulse Pressure					
PAP					
PAP MEAN					
LAP					
ICP					
	05/22/2006 10:12	05/22/2006 10:15	05/22/2006 11:37	05/22/2006 12:23	05/22/2006 12:51

Figure 8-2

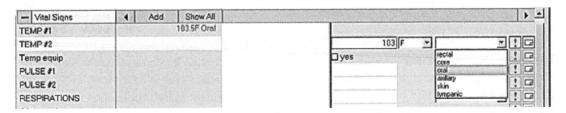

Figure 8-3

and time based on the current date and time. Always verify that this is the date and time when the vital signs were taken. There are scroll arrows that you can use to change it to the correct date and time.

Double clicking the name of the vital sign in the Vital Signs column opens an area of the chart where you can enter new values. You can enter a value or select a value from a drop-down list depending on the nature of the vital sign that you are entering into the chart.

Let's say that you are entering the patient's temperature for the second time in the day. Click TEMP#2 and it opens the temperature row in the chart. Type "103" and then open the next drop-down list to select "F" for Fahrenheit. The other option is Celsius. And then you select the last drop-down list box in that row to identify how the temperature was taken (Figure 8-3).

RED FLAG THE VITAL SIGNS

When a vital sign is significant, you should call it to the attention of other members of the healthcare team. This is easily accomplished using charting software because charting software has built-in flags to say, "Hey, take a look at this."

McKesson's charting software uses an exclamation mark as the red flag. Click the exclamation mark found at the right of the vital sign and the charting software displays the exclamation mark in red. Click the exclamation mark a second time to turn off the flag.

ENTERING COMMENTS

While turning on the exclamation mark calls attention to the vital sign, the healthcare team member must recognize the significance of the value. Many times this is obvious, such as a temperature of 103°F. Other times it is less obvious.

Take the patient's weight as an example. The patient's weight is entered into the computerized chart similar to temperature in that you enter the weight and corresponding metric such as ounces, kilogram, milligram, or gram. Suppose the weight changed significantly. This wouldn't be obvious even if the exclamation flag is turned on. The question is, what is the significance?

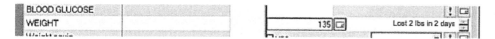

Figure 8-4

Charting software enables you to write a note explaining the significance. You open the note section by clicking an icon on the computerized chart. With McKesson's charting software, you click the icon to the right of the exclamation mark. This opens a text box where you can enter up to 255 characters. In our weight example, you might write "Lost 2 lbs in 2 days" (Figure 8-4).

Charting I&O

Charting software assures that I&O are calculated properly (as long as the correct amounts are entered into the chart) because the charting software does all of the math for you and displays the results on a summary screen.

You view the summary by clicking the I&O SUMMARY class in the left navigation panel (Figure 8-5). Displayed are total intake, total output, and the net value for each day and time that is charged.

Items are entered as volume or occurrences. A volume is a measurable amount of fluid and is measured in milliliters. An occurrence is fluid that is not measurable such as an apple. Only volume is included in the I&O calculation.

Below the summary section are an itemized list of intake and output charted. In this example, the nurse recorded the patient's intake at 10:12 on 5/22/2006 to be 50 mL of oral fluids, 8 mL of Ensure, and the patient's urine output was 25 mL.

Entering intake and output values is similar to the way you enter other vital signs into the chart. Click the appropriate class (Intake or Output) in the navigation bar to

		05/22/2006 10:12	05/22/2006 10:15	05/22/2006 11:37	05/22/2006 12:23	05/22/2006 12:51
ALL MEDS / Vital Signs	◄ ☐ More Results					►
I&O SUMMARY	─ IO SUMMARY ◄					►
INTAKE	Intake Total	58				525
OUTPUT	Output Total	25				550
	NET	33				-25
	─ INTAKE ◄ ⌁Chart					►
	Oral	50				400
	Ensure	8				
	Isocal					125
	Intake Total	58				525
	─ OUTPUT ◄ ⌁Chart					►
	Urine	25				550
	Output Total	25				550

Figure 8-5

display the page. The page contains a list of items that your healthcare facility wants measured. Double click the item and the charting software opens an area where you can enter a value.

Reviewing Your Entry

When you are finished updating the patient's chart, click the Save button. The Save button displays the Review page (Figure 8-6) where you give your entries a last look before they are saved to your patient's chart.

In this example, the temperature and weight that we entered are displayed, including the significance flag and the note that we wrote about the patient's weight.

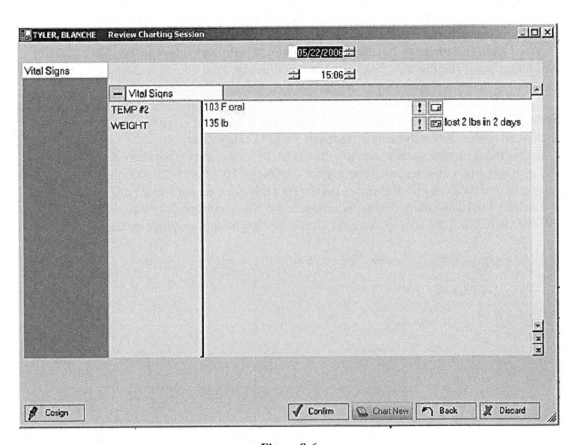

Figure 8-6

You are given four choices:

- Discard: The entry is erased and doesn't become part of your patient's chart.
- Back: Return to the chart to correct your entry.
- Chart New: Save your changes and chart a new patient.
- Confirm: Save your changes and continue to chart the current patient.

For example, after reviewing our charting you probably noticed that the significance flag for the patient's weight is not turned on, yet we noted that the patient lost 2 lbs in 2 days, which is probably significant. We could click the Back button and return to the weight entry to turn on the significance flag.

COSIGNING

Some entries must be cosigned by another member of the patient's healthcare team. This might be the case if the entry was made by a nursing assistant, who is authorized by the healthcare facility to update certain sections of the chart as long as the entry is cosigned by the patient's primary nurse.

Cosigning is also done electronically. McKesson's charting software enables a healthcare team member to cosign the Review screen by clicking the Cosign button where appropriate information is entered.

Most charting software prevents an entry that must be cosigned from being saved until the entry is cosigned. The charting software knows which activity and member of the healthcare team needs a cosigner by rights assigned to a healthcare team member's ID and a flag set on the activity in the charting software by the healthcare facility.

Summary

Charting software creates a To-Do List for a patient, your patients, or all the patients in your unit. The To-Do List tells what and when an activity needs to be performed along with display key information needed to perform the activity. Activities are also flagged overdue if it wasn't performed on time and STAT if the activity must be performed immediately.

Routine activities such as recording vital signs are entered in the vital signs portion of the computerized chart. Each vital sign is displayed in a table. Rows are types of vital signs and columns are date and time when the vital sign was assessed.

Vital signs are entered by typing its vital sign into the appropriate text box on the screen and then selecting a description of the vital sign from a drop-down list. Descriptions are usually defined by the healthcare facility.

You can highlight an entry if the vital sign value is significant by turning on a flag such as the exclamation mark in McKesson's software. The flag calls the attention of other members of the healthcare team to the vital sign. Likewise, you can insert a comment to describe the significance by entering a note alongside the vital sign.

Intake and output values are entered in the I&O section of the chart. The charting software list items that your healthcare facility wants charted, which are recorded as volume or occurrence. Charting software automatically calculates volume I&O values and displays them on the I&O Summary screen.

Charting software enables you to review your entry before saving it to the patient's chart. You are given the opportunity to discard your entry, change your entry, or save it. Furthermore, charting software provides a way for another member of the patient's healthcare team to cosign your entry.

Quiz

1. The date and time entered automatically by the charting software
   a. Is always correct because it is set by the IT department
   b. Must be reviewed and changed by the nurse if it is incorrect
   c. Must be reviewed and changed by the IT department if it is incorrect
   d. None of the above

2. Weight must be converted to pounds (lbs) in order for the weight to be entered into the chart.
   a. True
   b. False

3. The To-Do List displayed by charting software
   a. Is based on the charting software's assessment of which activity takes the longest to perform
   b. Is based on the date and time scheduled by the order
   c. Is based on the nurse manager's review of all activities for the unit
   d. Is based on the patient's medical diagnosis

4. The healthcare facility determines what items appear on the I&O page of the computerized chart.

   a. True

   b. False

5. You are limited to a 25-word comment for each vital sign entry.

   a. True

   b. False

6. If you discover an error in the Review page

   a. You can return to the chart without saving it and correct the error.

   b. Report the error to the nurse manager, who is authorized to correct the error.

   c. All error corrections must be electronically cosigned by the physician.

   d. None of the above.

7. You can request that the healthcare facility insert a new item to the I&O page.

   a. True

   b. False

8. With the To-Do List you can

   a. Display activity for only your patient

   b. Display activities for your patient that are overdue

   c. Display scheduled activities

   d. All of the above

9. Once you review and save your entries, they are immediately available to other members of the healthcare team.

   a. True

   b. False

10. The To-Do List contains the order number related to each activity that can be used to verify the order.

    a. True

    b. False

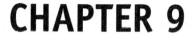

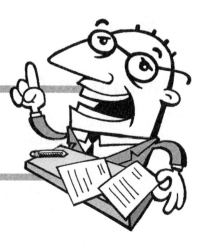

CHAPTER 9

Entering Patient Assessment in Charting Software

Chances are pretty good that if given a choice you would choose your cell phone over a land line in a blink of an eye. Both do the same thing, but the cell phone does it more efficiently. You'll have the same opinion about the ring binder chart after the first time you enter the results of your patient's assessment into charting software.

Charting software wins hands down because you can use charting software on a mobile computer at the patient's bedside to record your assessment results immediately as you assess your patient. Best of all, you can roll the mobile computer to assess your next patient without having to return to the nurses' station.

In this chapter, you'll build on your experience on how to enter vital signs from the previous chapter and learn how to enter assessment results in charting software.

Charting an Assessment

Your patient's computerized chart is divided into sections similar to the tabs in a ring binder chart. One of those sections is for documenting your assessment of the patient. The actual name of the section differs based on the charting software used by your healthcare facility. McKesson's charting software calls this the Assessment and Intervention section of their chart.

Once you open the section, usually by clicking the section tab, you'll see a clinical flow sheet. The clinical flow sheet lists the systems in the order in which it is assessed. McKesson refers to these items as classes. Typically, the clinical flow sheet begins with Neurological and continues in a top-down order that corresponds to the order in which you normally assess your patient. Think of the clinical flow sheet as a guide through your assessment.

Each class opens to a list of specific assessments. This is very similar to the vital signs section that you explored in Chapter 8 where each class opens a group of vital signs that you can review or enter into the patient's chart.

ENTERING AN ASSESSMENT

You'll see a list of assessments related to the class that you open when you double click on the class name. The actual items that you see depend on what charting software is used and possibly on the healthcare facility. Charting software manufacturers such as McKesson enables each healthcare facility to customize the list of assessment items.

In order to enter results of you assessment you must click the row containing the assessment. The charting software then opens the area where you can enter your assessment. This too is similar to how you displayed the area on the chart to enter vital signs.

PICK FROM A LIST

Charting software removes some ambiguities that commonly occur when charting an assessment in a ring binder chart. Instead of having to think of the right word to describe your assessment, charting software has a list of frequently used assessment results. You display the list and then pick the assessment result.

The list is usually a drop-down list that expands to show you all the options when you click the down arrow on the drop-down list. Items were selected for the list by the charting software manufacturer and by your healthcare facility, which means you're bound to find the proper description for your assessment on the list.

Let's say that you want to record your patient's level of consciousness. You'd click the Neurological class to display the list of neurological assessments

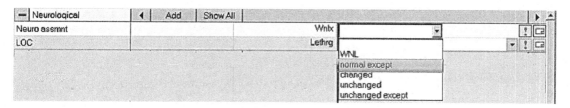

Figure 9-1

and then click the Neuro assmnt row to open the assessment area of the chart.

Clicking the arrow in the drop-down list box displays your choice of possible assessment results. If your patient is generally within normal range but there were some exceptions (Figure 9-1), you would select normal except. You can then note the exception in a comment (see Chapter 8).

MULTIPLE ASSESSMENTS

Many times the assessment results cannot be described in one word. For example, a patient may exhibit several signs that reflect the patient's level of consciousness. The manufacturers of charting software realize this and provide you with a list of check boxes with each check box representing an assessment result.

You are probably familiar with how to use check boxes because they are widely used in software that you use on your home computer. Click the check box once and a check appears indicating that the item is selected. Click the check box again and the check is removed from the check box, indicating that the item is no longer selected.

Each section of the electronic chart is jam-packed with information about the patient. Since space in the section is at a premium, the folks who design charting software typically use one line per assessment item, which doesn't leave room for a bunch of check boxes.

McKesson's designers managed to accommodate multiple assessments by incorporating check boxes in a drop-down list. Click the drop-down list to display multiple assessments and then click away from the drop-down list and the drop-down list collapses into a single line on the chart.

PICKING MULTIPLE ASSESSMENTS

Suppose you want to enter an assessment of your patient's level of consciousness. First you would click the LOC line in the Neurological class and then click the drop-down list. The drop-down list contains a list of assessment results, each as a check box (Figure 9-2).

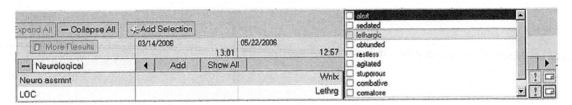

Figure 9-2

These include

- Alert
- Sedated
- Lethargic
- Obtunded
- Restless
- Agitated
- Stuporous
- Combative
- Comatose

Click the appropriate check boxes. If you click one in error, simply click it again to remove the check mark. When you're finished entering your LOC assessment, click outside the drop-down list to close it.

CONSOLIDATING YOUR ASSESSMENT

When your assessment response entails multiple assessment results, charting software consolidates your multiple results and displays it on the row that contains your assessment. This makes it easy for other members of the healthcare team to quickly review your assessment.

Say that your patient is gasping and grunting when you performed the sound/breathing portion of the Respiratory assessment. You document your findings by clicking the sound/breathing row to open its drop-down list. Select Gasping and then select Grunting. Chart software automatically combines these and displays them on the row (Figure 9-3).

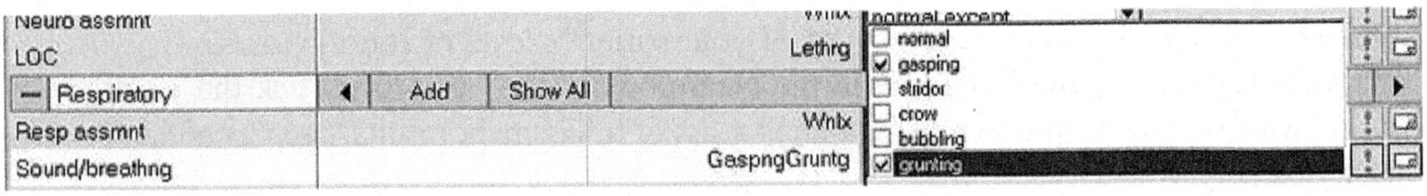

Figure 9-3

SOMETHING UNUSUAL

If words you pick from the drop-down list don't fully convey the condition of your patient, you can elaborate by entering a comment. As you'll remember from the previous chapter, a comment can be up to 255 characters that is directly associated with each item on the chart.

In McKesson's software, click the rightmost icon in the row to open the comment text box and then begin typing your note. Click elsewhere on the chart to resume charting. Click on the comment icon again to see and modify the comment.

If the assessment result is unusual and should be reviewed by other members of the healthcare team, then set the urgent flag to on. The exclamation mark icon in McKesson's charting software is the urgent flag. Click it to set the urgent flag on and click it again to turn off the urgent flag.

SAVING AND REVIEWING

When you are finished entering your assessment results in the chart, click Save at the bottom of the chart. This displays the Review screen, which is similar to the Review screen you learned to use in Chapter 8.

You'll recall that you can select

- Discard: The entry is erased and doesn't become part of your patient's chart.
- Back: Return to the chart to correct your entry.
- Chart New: Save your changes and chart a new patient.
- Confirm: Save your changes and continue to chart the current patient.

Summary

Patient assessments are recorded in the assessment section of the computerized chart. The actual name of the section is unique to the charting software and in some instances unique to the healthcare facility.

The assessment section is organized in a clinical flow sheet that corresponds to the clinical flow used to assess a patient. Each system is identified as a class within the clinical flow and within each class are assessments.

The result of an assessment is documented by clicking the corresponding row of the assessment and then entering the results in the charting software. Results are entered by selecting one or more words from the assessment's drop-down list. Multiple selections are recorded by clicking the appropriate check boxes on the list.

Once the assessment is entered, click Save to display the Review screen where you can verify your results and save them to the computerized chart, modify them, or discard the results.

Quiz

1. The clinical flow sheet is
   a. A printed copy of your assessment.
   b. Used to cosign an assessment electronically.
   c. The order in which the assessment is listed in charting software.
   d. None of the above.

2. To elaborate on an assessment you would
   a. Add a comment to the assessment.
   b. Turn on the urgent flag.
   c. Notify each member of the healthcare team individually.
   d. Notify each member of the healthcare team with an email blast.

3. If you selected the wrong word on the drop-down list in your assessment, you
   a. Enter a comment.
   b. Click the urgent flag.
   c. Click the word or check box to unselect it.
   d. None of the above.

4. Notify the person in your healthcare facility who is responsible for charting software if you want to add an assessment description to a drop-down list.
   a. True
   b. False

5. You can review the history of a patient's assessments by scrolling through the patient's chart.
   a. True
   b. False

6. The nurse must
   a. Review assessment results entered into charting software before saving it.
   b. Correct errors in the assessment result immediately.

c.   Flag unexpected results as urgent.

   d.   All of the above.

7. You should never record the results of your patient assessment at the bedside using charting software

   a.   True

   b.   False

8. Once you save your assessment results in charting software

   a.   The patient's family can review the chart using their Internet connection.

   b.   The healthcare team can review the chart anywhere within the healthcare facility's computer network.

   c.   The patient can review his or her chart online.

   d.   None of the above.

9. The nurse manager can review your assessment results without having to notify you.

   a.   True

   b.   False

10. Healthcare facilities provide training to employees on using charting software.

   a.   True

   b.   False

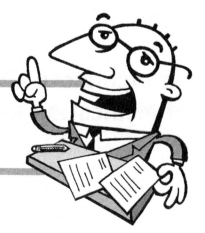

CHAPTER 10

Entering Medication Administration Charting Software

Errors can easily occur when administrating medication to your patient because there are possible gaps in communication among the physician who orders the medication, the pharmacist who provides it, and the nurse who administers the medication to the patient.

Charting software greatly reduces the risk for errors by providing a clear channel for communication among the healthcare team and by applying built-in controls in the software to automatically enforce the five rights of medication administration.

In this chapter, you will learn how these built-in controls work and how to use the charting software to administer and document medication that you give to your patient.

Enforcing the Five Rights of Medication Administration

Your instructor probably never let you forget the five rights of medication administration. These rights guarantee the patient that

- The right medication is administered
- To the right patient
- At the right time
- In the right dose
- Using the right route

Charting software automates this process by using bar codes to identify the patient and the medication, then comparing the medication and the current time with the medication order to assure that the five rights of medication administration are being followed.

The patient's wrist band has a bar code that translates into the patient's ID. The wrist band also contains the patient's ID and other information in a format that you can easily read. A handheld bar code reader that is attached to the computer is focused on the patient's wrist band (Figure 10-1). Pressing the button on the bar code reader causes a red light to shine on the wrist band, which reads the bar code and beeps when it is finished reading it.

The medication label also has a bar code (Figure 10-2) that identifies the medication, dose, route, and the patient who should receive the medication. This is in addition to the same information in a form that you can read without using the bar code reader. The bar code on the medication label is scanned similar to how the patient's wrist band is scanned.

Once both the patient's ID and the medication ID are read, the charting software retrieves the patient's medication administration record, the medication order written by the physician, and medication information entered by the pharmacist.

Inside the computer, a number of things happen.

- The current date and time are compared to the date and time that medication is scheduled to be administered. This assures that the medication is being administered at the proper time.

- The medication is compared to medications that were already administered to the patient. This determines if the patient already received the scheduled medication and thereby prevents the patient from receiving a second dose.

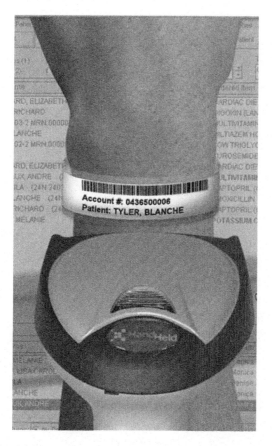

Figure 10-1   Aim the bar code reader at the patient's wrist band and press the button to read the bar code into the charting software.

- The medication, dose, and route are compared to the medication order written by the physician to determine if the medication that is at bedside conforms to the medication order.

- The medication is compared to other medications that the patient was recently administered to identify contraindications. For example, the medication may have to be given at least an hour after other medication was administered to the patient. The charting software will detect if an hour has passed.

A warning message is displayed on the computer if the charting software detects that any of the five rights of medication administration is being violated. If no violations occur, then the charting software automatically displays the patient's medication record on the screen.

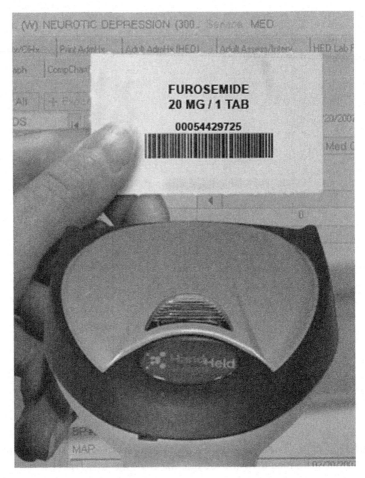

Figure 10-2   Aim the bar code reader at the bar code on the medication label then press the button to read the bar code into the charting software.

The Workflow

It is important to keep in mind that charting software is a tool that helps reduce risks associated with administering medication to your patient. It is not a substitute for following standard medication administration procedures.

The workflow for medication administration is the same regardless of if charting software is used to assist you. You begin by reviewing the medication order. The medication order appears on the patient's electronic chart. The medication order is entered into the charting software either by the physician or by the nurse under the physician's direction. You will see how this is done in Chapter 11.

Once the medication order is reviewed, you will need to collect the medication, which is usually from the medication room in the unit. Depending on the nature of the medication, the route used, and how the medication is provided by the pharmacy, you may have to prepare the medication in the medication room.

Next, take the medication to the bedside. Before administering the medication to your patient, you must verify that you have the right patient, the right medication, the right dose, the right time, and the right route.

This is where the workflow differs slightly from times when charting software isn't used for medication administration. Instead of reading the patient's wrist band yourself, you scan the patient's bar code into the charting software, which displays the patient's chart.

HINT *It is always a good idea to compare information displayed on the patient's chart with the information on the patient's wrist band to make sure that you have the right patient.*

After verifying the patient, the bar code on the medication is scanned into the charting software. This causes the charting software to open areas on the chart where you can enter information about how the medication was administered. You will learn more about this in the next section when you walk through the process of documenting medication that is administered to the patient. Some charting software may require that the medication bar code be scanned twice as a check and balance to assure that the medication is correct for the patient per the medication order.

Next, give the medication to the patient. Charting software gives you a place to enter comments alongside the medication in the chart such as how well the patient accepted the medication.

The last step is to select the Confirm button on the charting software indicating that you are finished administering medication to the patient. This causes the charting software to save the medication record to the patient's chart. Once saved, this information is available to members of the patient's healthcare team from computers on the hospital's computer network.

Using Charting Software to Document Medication Administration

Now that you have an understanding of how charting software is used to document medication administration, let's walk through the processing using McKesson's charting software. Although your healthcare facility may use different charting software, it is likely to work similar to McKesson's charting software.

Medical Charting Demystified

Patient Name	Scheduled	Group	Status	Ordered Item	Dose/Duration	Route	Prty Freq (Rate)	Order #'s
TYLER, BLANCHE	02/21 08:00	MEDS	Scheduled	FUROSEMIDE	20 MG=1 TAB	ORAL	RTN BIDBL	7734 (4)
24N 2402-2 MRN:00000106	02/21 10:00	MEDS	Scheduled	DILTIAZEM HCL (CARDIZEM SR)	90 MG=1 CP12	ORAL	RTN Q12H	7733 (3)
	02/21 12:00	DTY	Scheduled	LOW TRIGLYCERIDE			DTY TIMED MEALS	2359966
		MEDS	Scheduled	FUROSEMIDE	20 MG=1 TAB	ORAL	RTN BIDBL	7734 (4)
	02/21 14:00	MEDS	Scheduled	AMOXICILLIN (AMOXIL)	500 MG=1 CAP	ORAL	RTN Q8H	7716 (1)
	-----------	MEDS	PRN	ACETAMINOPHEN	650 MG=(2 x 325 MG TA	ORAL	PRN Q6HP	7732 (2)

Figure 10-3   The charting software automatically displays the patient's medication orders once the patient's bar code is scanned into the software.

You've been assigned to Blanche Tyler. It is 7:50 a.m. and you review Ms. Tyler's chart and notice that she is to receive furosemide 20-mg tablet at 8 a.m. The status is Scheduled, which indicates that she has not received the medication as yet.

First, you get the medication from the medication room. Since this is a tablet, there is no medication preparation required. You return to the patient's bedside and then scan the patient's bar code into the charting software. The charting software displays Ms. Tyler's medication orders (Figure 10-3).

Scan the bar code on the furosemide label. This causes a medication administration entry to open in Ms. Tyler's chart. By default, the charting software displays the name of the medication, the dose, and route to be used. In this example, the medication ordered is 20 mg per tablet to be administered orally.

The charting software enables you to overwrite the dose and number of tablets because the pharmacy might have delivered a different dose per tablet (Figure 10-4). For example, the pharmacy might have delivered 10 mg per tablet. This means that the patient receives two tablets of 10 mg tablets rather than one 20-mg tablet. This complies with the medication order; however, you must overwrite the default values displayed by the charting software to reflect medication that was administered to the patient.

In the upper right corner of Figure 10-4 is an envelope icon. As you will recall from previous chapters, selecting this icon displays a note pad where you can enter a comment. A comment reflects something unusual that occurred when trying to administer this medication to the patient such as the patient refusal to take the medication.

An exclamation mark appears to the left of the comment icon. This is selected if you want to call the comment to the attention of other members of the healthcare team. It suggests that you better take a look at this!

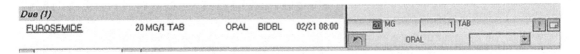

Figure 10-4   Fields are opened automatically when you scan the medication bar code, enabling you to overwrite default values and enter comments.

The number and types of fields that are available to document the medication administration varies depending on the nature of the medication and the medication order. For example, you won't see a field for pump setting unless the medication is being administered IV.

HINT *Always notify the physician personally whenever a problem arises when administering medication to the patient. Don't simply enter a comment and set the exclamation mark on.*

Scan the medication's bar code again and the charting software displays a preview of information that will be recorded in the patient's chart. This reflects any changes that you made to the entry in the previous screen. Don't do anything with this screen.

Now it is time to administer the furosemide to Ms. Tyler. If all goes well, you can select the Confirm button on the bottom of the screen (Figure 10-5). This saves the information. You're finished.

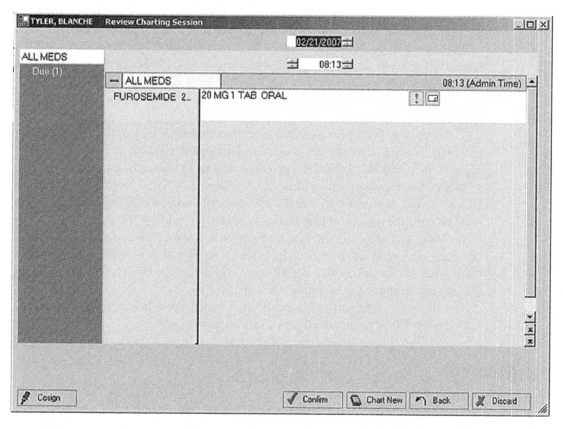

Figure 10-5   Select Confirm to document that you administered medication to Ms. Tyler.

However, if something noteworthy occurs such as Ms. Tyler refusing to take the medication, then you can Select the Back button to return to the previous screen where you can enter a comment and change other information associated with administering medication to Ms. Tyler. If you do this, you will need to scan the medication bar code once you are finished changing the information in the charting software.

Recovering When Things Go Wrong

Although computer technology has its benefits such as providing reliable checks and balances when administering medication, there are occasions when technology fails to operate as planned. This is true about charting software. Fortunately, designers of charting software offer a built-in work around when failure occurs.

A common failure with charting software is when the bar code reader is unable to read the patient's bar code as a result of wear and tear on the patient's wrist band. This is especially true if the patient is admitted to the healthcare facility for a long stay. Rarely does this happen with bar codes on medications because the bar code and label are printed within hours of the medication being administered to the patient.

There are two ways to notice when the bar code reader fails to read the patient's bar code. First, you don't hear a beep when scanning the bar code. The beep signals that the bar code is successfully read. No beep tells you there is a problem. When this happens you can reposition the wrist band in front of the bar code reader or wipe the bar code reader to remove any dust that may block the scan.

The other way you know there is a problem scanning is by looking at the charting software. If after scanning the patient's chart doesn't appear or the wrong chart appears, then you know there is a problem reading the patient's bar code.

When this happens, you will need to order a new wrist band for the patient. However, you still must administer the patient's administration. Therefore, you must retrieve the patient's chart manually using the charting software.

Let's say you are administering medication to Richard Blaney and Mr. Blaney's bar code isn't read by the bar code reader. The first step is to find Mr. Blaney's chart. With McKesson's charting software you Select the HED tab and then Select Mr. Blaney from the list of patients (Figure 10-6).

Mr. Blaney's chart shows his medication order. From this point, you continue with the workflow as described previously in this chapter.

Summary

Charting software reduces the risk of errors that occur when administering medication to patients by providing an automatic check and balance and by enforcing the five rights of medication administration.

Notify	Last	First	Dept	Rm/Bed	Diagnosis		Gen..	MRN
0	DANIELS	MELANIE	24N	2400-1	(W) ABDOMINAL PAIN UNSPEC..		F	000001055
1	FREMONT	LISA CAROL	24N	2401-1	(W) PATHOLOGIC FX,UNSPEC..		F	000001060
2	CRANE	LILA	24N	2402-1	(W) OTALGIA NOS (388.70)		F	000001056
3	TYLER	BLANCHE	24N	2402-2	(W) NEUROTIC DEPRESSION (..		F	000001065
4	DEVEREAUX	ANDRE	24N	2403-1	(W) CHEST PAIN NOS (786.50)		M	000001052
5	BLANEY	RICHARD	24N	2403-2	(W) FEVER (780.6)		M	000001051
6	LUMLEY	GEORGE	24N	2404-1	(W) CHEST PAIN NOS (786.50)		M	000001050
7	OACKLEY	CHARLIE	24N	2406-1	(W) GASTROINTEST HEMORR..		M	000001061
8	EVERGUARD	ELIZABETH	24N	2409-1	(W) TACHYCARDIA NOS (785.0)		F	000001121
9								

Figure 10-6   Select the patient's chart manually if the bar code reader fails to read the patient's bar code.

You follow basically the same workflow when using charting software as you do if charts are kept in a binder. That is, check the patient's chart for medication; prepare the medication; bring the medication to the bedside; verify the patient, medication, dose, route, and time; administer the medication; and then document.

The patient's wrist band and the medication label contain a bar code that is scanned into the charting software using a bar code reader. The bar code uniquely identifies the patient and the medication and is used by the charting software to display the appropriate section of the patient's chart that pertains to administering the medication.

Once these bar codes are scanned, charting software verifies the accuracy of the information by comparing it to the medication order that the physician entered into the charting software. Any discrepancies cause the charting software to signal an error on the screen and prevent you from proceeding.

If the bar code reader is unable to read a bar code, you must then display the patient's chart manually using charting software.

Quiz

1. A bar code

   a. Is a series of dark bars of various thicknesses that represents a unique number

   b. Consists of the patient's first and last name, place of birth, and next of kin

   c. Consists of the day and time that the medication should be administered to the patient

   d. None of the above

2. If the patient refuses to take the medication, then
   a. Enter a comment in the charting software and set the exclamation flag.
   b. Notify the physician personally, enter a comment in the charting software, and set the exclamation flag.
   c. Notify the nurse manager.
   d. None of the above.

3. Once you document that you administered medication to the patient using charting software,
   a. Any member of the healthcare team can access the medication record from within the healthcare facility's computer network.
   b. Any member of the healthcare team can access the medication records only from the computer at your nurse's station.
   c. Any member of the healthcare team can access the medication records only from the mobile computer that you used to update the patient chart at the patient's bedside.
   d. None of the above.

4. Charting software automatically checks the five rights of medication administration.
   a. True
   b. False

5. Information displayed by charting software is always correct.
   a. True
   b. False

6. If the pharmacy delivered medication that was 30 mg per tablet and the charting software showed 15-mg tablets, you would
   a. Call the physician to have the medication order changed.
   b. Call the pharmacy to have the correct dose delivered.
   c. Overwrite the values displayed by the charting software.
   d. None of the above.

7. If the bar code reader is unable to read the patient's bar code, then manually display the patient's chart.
   a. True
   b. False

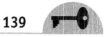

8. If the medication scheduled in the charting software isn't in the medication room, then

    a.   Assume that the medication order was cancelled.

    b.   Call the pharmacy and ask that they deliver the medication.

    c.   Call the physician to confirm that the order was cancelled.

    d.   None of the above.

9. If you suspect that the scheduled medication shown in charting software is contraindicated for your patient, then call the physician immediately.

    a.   True

    b.   False

10. You are prohibited from changing information displayed in the medication administration area of the patient's electronic chart.

    a.   True

    b.   False

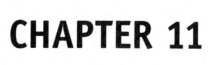

CHAPTER 11

Entering Orders in Charting Software

A key component of charting software is a feature that enables physicians and other members of the healthcare team to enter orders into the patient's chart. An order directs one or more members of the healthcare team to perform a test, administer a treatment, or do something that will help restore the patient's health.

Although physicians enter orders directly into charting software, there are times when orders are entered by the nurse on behalf of the physician. And depending on the policy of the healthcare facility, the nurse may be authorized to write some orders directly.

This chapter shows you how to enter orders into charting software.

An Order

A patient is a puzzle for the healthcare team to solve. The patient arrives at the healthcare facility reporting symptoms that are subjective based on the patient's perception. Some symptoms are clues to the puzzle, wheras other symptoms are unrelated. The healthcare team then looks for signs, which are objective clues that point to disease.

The combination of symptoms and signs typically raises suspicion as to the underlying problem, but not enough information to solve the puzzle. Suspicion enables the healthcare team to further explore the patient's condition using medical tests.

A medical test can involve analyzing bodily fluid or looking inside the patient using x-rays, magnetic resonance imaging (MRI), or in extreme situations surgically entering the body to remove samples such as biopsy material.

Since the patient's primary physician doesn't personally perform these tests, the physician writes an order directing that other members of the healthcare team to perform the tests and report their findings to the physician. The findings are additional clues help the physician and other members of the healthcare team diagnose the patient's problem.

Once a diagnosis is made, the physician determines a course of treatment that is expected to restore the patient's health. The treatment may involve medication, therapy, or in extreme situations surgery. The patient's primary physician writes an order directing that other members of the healthcare team to treat the patient.

A healthcare facility might have a policy of standing orders. A standing order specifies a pattern of facts that if exists authorizes the nurse to write a specific order for the patient without obtaining permission from the patient's primary physician.

For example, a standing order might exist directing the nurse to order a pregnancy test for female patients before administering medication that is contraindicated for pregnancy. Likewise, there might be a standing order that all patients who are admitted to the healthcare facility receive a series of screening laboratory tests as a precaution. Once the physician admits the patient, the nurse then writes the order for the lab tests.

Entering the Order

The first step in entering a new order is to display the patient's chart. As you learned in previous chapters, you select the patient's name from the census to display the patient's chart using McKesson's charting software. This is similar to how you display a chart using other charting software.

In this example, Blanche Tyler is the patient, and by selecting her name the charting software displays a listing of current orders for this patient (Figure 11-1). At the top of the screen is the New Order button. Select it to enter a new order for the patient.

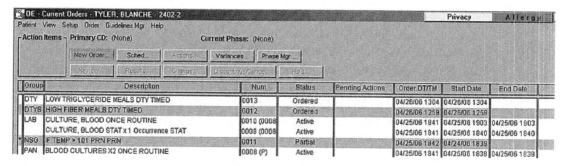

Figure 11-1   At the top of the Current Order screen is the New Order button. Select the New Order button to write a new order for your patient.

As you can imagine, there are hundreds of different kinds of orders that can be written for a patient. Charting software uses various techniques to make it easy to find the order that you want to enter for the patient.

After selecting the New Order button, the Order Selection screen displays. The Order Selection screen is used to locate the type of order that you want to write. The trick to quickly finding the order among the hundreds of orders in the charting software is to know the code of the order group that contains the order.

An order group is a collection of related orders such as lab, dietary, and radiology. Depending on the charting software, groups are defined by either the software manufacturer or by the healthcare facility, which is the case with McKesson's charting software.

Each order group is assigned a code such as:

CONS = Consult

DYT = Dietary

ED = Education

LAB = Lab

NSG = Nursing

RAD = Radiology

WEIG = Weigh

The group code is also referred to as an alias. You enter the name of the order or the group code in the Search By box in the upper left order of the Order Selection screen or simply click the group in the Search Categories box. Select the Find button and the Charting software displays a list of orders that are associated with that order group.

Let's say that Blanche Tyler's primary physician asked you to enter an order to have Ms. Tyler weighed every day. Based on the order groups supplied to you by the healthcare facility, you know that WEIG is the group code for weight-related orders. You enter WEIG into the Search By box and click Find. The list of weigh orders appears in the Order Options box (Figure 11-2).

There are four orders listed in the weight group. If there were more orders than can be displayed in the Order Options box, then you would see a vertical scroll bar appear that would enable you to scroll down the list.

Next, highlight the order that you wish to write and click the Select button. The Select button tells the charting software to copy the order to the Selected Orders box. The Selected Orders box lists orders that you are writing.

HINT *You can select more than one order from the list by holding down the Ctrl button when highlighting the order.*

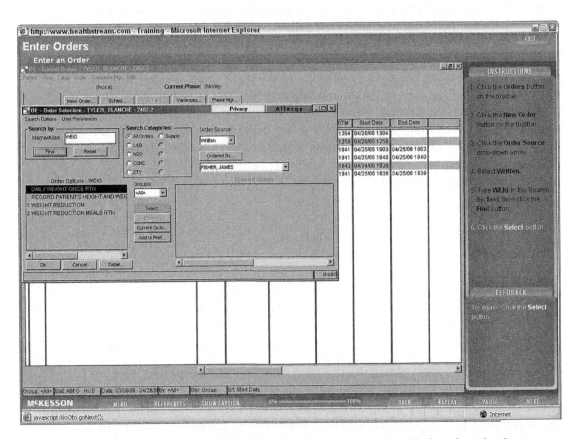

Figure 11-2 The Order Options box lists all orders that are associated with the selected order group.

HOW WAS IT WRITTEN?

You will need to identify the Order Source by entering the source in the top right corner of the Order Selection screen. The Order Source describes how the order is communicated. You select the Order Source from the Order Source drop-down list.

There are four types of order sources: written, verbal, telephone, and direct.

Written

A written order is an order where the physician literally writes the order into the patient's paper chart. Typically, this occurs during the period when the healthcare facility is transitioning from paper to electronic charts. The nurse must transcribe the written order into the electronic order.

Verbal

A verbal order is an order given by the physician to the nurse. This commonly occurs when both the physician and the nurse are at the patient's bedside or during daily rounds.

Telephone

A telephone order is similar to a verbal order except that the physician places the order with the nurse over the telephone. This happens frequently when the nurse calls the physician to report the results of a test and the physician orders a follow-up test or treatment.

Direct

A direct order is an order entered by the physician or the authorized member of the healthcare team.

WHO WROTE THE ORDER?

You must specify who wrote the order by entering the healthcare team member's name in the Ordered By box that is below the Order Source box in the top right corner of the Order Selection screen. Some charting software, including McKesson's, refers to the person who writes the order as the provider.

Depending on the charting software used by your healthcare facility and by the healthcare facility's policy, you may see a drop-down list of providers. The drop-down list typically lists the patient's primary physician, attending physician, or providers who have written orders for the patient. Furthermore, the patient's primary physician might be chosen as the default for the new order and appears automatically in the Ordered By box. In this example, James Fisher is Ms. Tyler's primary physician.

Although setting a default provider is a time-saving feature, it is also risky because an assumption might be made that the default provider is writing the order when, in fact, the order is written by a different provider. Therefore, some healthcare facilities may not set a default provider nor provide a list of providers who most frequently write orders for the patient.

If the provider's name doesn't appear in the drop-down list box or if there isn't a list or default provider, then you must search from among all providers who are associated with the healthcare facility. You do this by clicking the Ordered By button.

Selecting the Ordered By button causes the Staff Select screen to appear (Figure 11-3). This is where you locate the provider who is writing the order. You can imagine this is like trying to find a needle in a haystack; however, charting software has a few shortcuts to make your search easy.

You can limit your search to a particular group of staff by selecting the group from the Group drop-down list that appears on the left side of the screen. Likewise, you can limit the search to a specific facility by picking the facility from the Facility drop-down list located below the Group drop-down list.

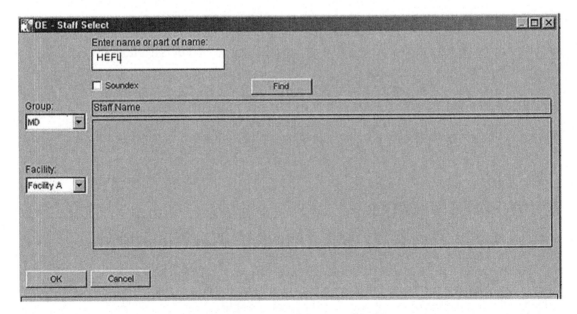

Figure 11-3   Speed your search by selecting groups of staff to search rather than searching the entire list of employees.

Enter the full or partial name of the provider in the box at the top of the screen and then click the Find button. The charting software displays every staff member that matches the search criteria. Highlight the name and select OK to enter the provider in the order.

HINT *Let's say that you're unsure of spelling, but you can phonically spell the name. Select the Soundex box and then enter the phonic spelling of the provider in the search criteria and then select the Find button. The charting software searches the staff for names that phonically match the search criteria.*

ORDER DETAILS

After selecting the order from the list of orders, you will need to enter details of the order. You do this by selecting the Details button on the bottom of the Order Selection screen. The Details button opens the Order Detail screen (Figure 11-4).

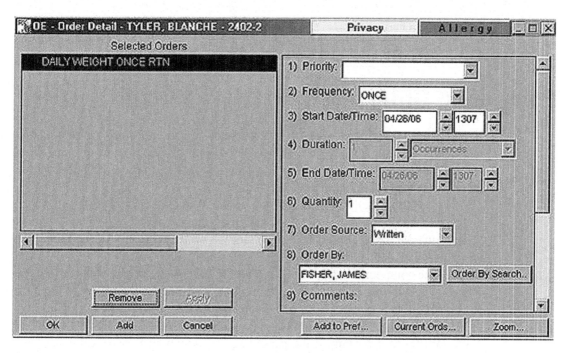

Figure 11-4 Highlight the order, enter details, and then select OK to save the order to the patient's chart.

The Order Detail screen displays a list of selected orders on the right side of the screen. In this example, there is only one order, which is daily weight for Ms. Tyler. Additional orders would appear if multiple orders were selected.

Highlight an order and the charting software displays details that are associated with the order. Types of details will differ depending on the nature of the order.

Some details such as start date and time and frequency are filled in for you. These are referred to as default settings. You must verify that these settings are correct and change them if necessary.

Other details are blank requiring you to enter information. You do this by selecting a choice from a drop-down menu or using up and down arrows to change the value displayed on the screen, as is the case with Quantity.

Still other details are grayed, prohibiting you from changing the value. Charting software grays a value for one of three reasons. First, the value cannot be changed until you enter a previous value. Once the previous value is entered, charting software ungrays the value, enabling you to change it. Another reason for graying a value is because the value is set by default. For example, if frequency is set to Once, the duration must be 1. Or the charting software determined that the detail does not pertain to the order.

Also on the Order Detail screen you can select the Remove button to remove the order, select the Add button to insert a new order, or select OK to save the order to the patient's chart.

Compound Order

A compound order is an order that consists of two or more other orders and is identified by a unique name. A complete blood count (CBC) is an example. CBC is a group of blood tests that is commonly ordered together to provide the healthcare team with glimpse into the patient's health.

The healthcare facility or the charting software manufacturer defines groups of tests based on the policy of the healthcare facility and defines the group code, or alias, to the compound order. You then enter the group code, or alias, as the search criteria to display the compound order.

Once the compound order is selected, the charting software compares orders that make up the compound order with orders already written for the patient in an effort to prevent duplicate orders from being entered.

For example, a physician might have previously written an order for a white blood count (WBC) to determine if the patient has an infection. Subsequently, an order might be written for a CBC, which is a compound order that contains a WBC.

Rather than automatically processing the CBC order, the charting software searches previous orders to determine if the WBC had been ordered. If so, then the charting software either removes the WBC from the CBC order or enters a comment on the CBC order that the WBC was already ordered depending on the type of charting software being used.

Summary

Charting software enables the physician or other member of the healthcare team to enter orders directly into the patient's electronic chart. Once entered, the member of the healthcare team who is responsible for carrying out the order receives the order electronically and then documents the result after the order is performed.

To enter a new order, display the patient's chart then open a new order screen. Each order is assigned to a group of related orders called an Order Group, which is identified by a group code. The group code used as the search criteria causes the charting software to display a listing of orders assigned to the group.

Highlight the order(s) on the list and click the Select button to select the order. Click the Details button to enter details of the order. The type of details will differ depending on the nature of the order.

For each order you need to select the Order Source, which is how the order was communicated to the person entering the order into the charting software. You also need to enter the name of the provider who is writing the order. You pick the provider's name from a list of staff that appears in the charting software.

Once all the information is entered, select the OK button and the order is saved to the patient's chart.

Quiz

1. The patient's complaint is referred to as
   a. A sign
   b. A symptom
   c. An issue
   d. None of the above
2. A standing order is
   a. An order that appears in an Order Group.
   b. An order that is common among all healthcare facilities.

c. An order that specifies a pattern of facts that if it exists authorizes the nurse to write a specific order for the patient without obtaining permission from the patient's primary physician.

   d. None of the above.

3. A provider is considered

   a. All members of the healthcare team.

   b. All members of the healthcare team for a particular patient.

   c. A member of the healthcare team who is authorized to write an order.

   d. None of the above.

4. Charting software automatically checks to see if orders in a compound order have been previously written for the patient.

   a. True

   b. False

5. Charting software enables you to locate a provider by using phonic spelling.

   a. True

   b. False

6. A detail of an order is grayed because

   a. Another detail must be entered before entering the detail that is grayed.

   b. The detail value is set by default based on a value of another detail.

   c. The detail does not pertain to the order.

   d. All of the above.

7. You can select more than one order from the Order Group by holding down the Ctrl key when highlighting the order.

   a. True

   b. False

8. If the physician gives you an order at the patient's bedside during morning rounds, you would identify the source of order as

   a. Verbal

   b. Direct

   c. Written

   d. None of the above

9. A telephone order is recorded as a verbal order.

   a.   True

   b.   False

10. Your healthcare facility provides you with a list of group codes that identify groups of orders.

   a.   True

   b.   False

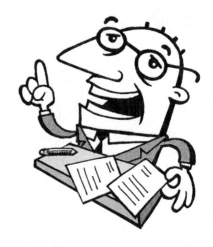

Final Exam

1. A new nurse tells you that she helped a patient back to bed after he slipped putting on his slippers. What is the best response?

    a. Report the nurse to your supervisor.

    b. Write an incident report.

    c. Ask the nurse to write an incident report.

    d. Thank the nurse for helping the patient.

2. The nurse auscultates rales in the base of her patient's left lung. Which part of the care map/care plan will you document that information?

    a. Assessment

    b. Diagnosis

    c. Intervention

    d. Evaluation

3. Patient information is stored electronically in multiple places.

    a. True

    b. False

4. The To-Do List displayed by charting software

   a. Is based on the charting software's assessment of which activity takes the longest to perform

   b. Is based on the date and time scheduled by the order

   c. Is based on the nurse manager's review of all activities for the unit

   d. None of the above

5. A computerized chart

   a. Cannot be accessed by the patient's primary physician

   b. Cannot be accessed using a mobile computer on the unit

   c. Is stored in multiple locations

   d. None of the above.

6. The best way to envision a computer network is as

   a. A cable

   b. A complex series of wires

   c. As your hometown

   d. As wifi

7. Your patient is a 72-year-old man who is 12 hours' a postop following an open cholescystectomy. Your report from the previous nurse indicated the following: alert and oriented × 3; pleasant, cooperative, and appropriate; surgical dressing dry and intact; vital signs WNL; pain level 2/10 as per pain scale. When you evaluate the patient for your a.m. assessment, he calls you by his daughter's name, shows facial grimacing with incisional palpation, unable to describe pain level, and tells you that he is late for work. What would you write in his chart?

   a. Alert and oriented, denies pain, agree with previous assessment.

   b. Confusion to place

   c. Alert, disoriented to place, responses inappropriate, demonstrates facial grimacing with incisional palpation, pain level indeterminable

   d. None of the above

8. The best way to avoid errors when updating the MAR is to

   a. Use abbreviates adopted by your healthcare facility

   b. Update the MAR immediately after you administer medication to a patient

   c. Dropping the zero following the decimal

   d. All of the above

9. After leaving the patient's room, the physician tells you that the patient is DNR. An hour later, the patient goes into cardiac arrest. The best response is to:

   a. Don't call a code

   b. Call a code

   c. Determine if the physician has written a DNR order

   d. Call a slow code

10. The medical laboratory has to be informed of medication given to the patient immediately prior to taking a blood sample.

    a. True

    b. False

11. Which of the following should be removed from the chart?

    a. Care plan

    b. Medical insurance information

    c. Opinions from a specialist who review test results

    d. An incident report

12. What is the best form used to record the amount of IV fluid that was given to a patient?

    a. Transfer form

    b. Intake and Output form

    c. Progress notes

    d. KARDEX

13. Patient information entered into charting software is stored in a router.

    a. True

    b. False

14. A computerized chart can be

    a. Reviewed simultaneously by different members of the healthcare team on different computers

    b. Restricted according to rights set by the IT department according to the healthcare facility's policies

    c. Be accessed by the patient's primary nurse

    d. All of the above

15. The To-Do List generated by charting software contains the patient name related to each activity that can be used to verify the order.

   a. True

   b. False

16. Encryption is

   a. Converting information into meaningless information using a key and mathematical formula

   b. Used to validate your user ID when logging into the computer

   c. Used by the network administrator to reject invalid log user IDs

   d. All of the above

17. The nurse is caring for a patient with orthostatic hypotension. The nurse's assessment concurs with that diagnosis. The most accurate documentation of that assessment is.

   a. Patient appears to be dizzy when standing.

   b. Patient complains of dizziness while ambulating.

   c. Patient's blood pressure lying down is 148/86; when patient stands at bedside, blood pressure is 132/70.

   d. a.m. assessment BP 150/92.

18. When is the most appropriate time to modify a care plan?

   a. Never

   b. Upon readmission

   c. Following assessment of the patient

   d. At the request of the physician

19. The best way to think of a DBMS is as an electronic filing cabinet and super–file clerk.

   a. True

   b. False

20. Once logged into the computer, the access granted to the ID changes depending on who is using the computer.

   a. True

   b. False

21. You are limited to a 255-word comment for each vital sign entry.

   a. True

   b. False

22. The day nurse charts for his end of shift note that the patient is lethargic. The night nurse expects to find the patient:

    a. Fast asleep

    b. Awake, alert, and oriented

    c. Sleepy but arousable

    d. Confused and disoriented

23. Who can not modify a care plan?

    a. The charge nurse

    b. The nursing assistant

    c. The LPN

    d. The primary nurse

24. You are supervising a student nurse who makes an error when charting progress notes. What should you do?

    a. Explain that errors occur and then draw a single line through the error and initial it.

    b. Explain that errors occur and give the nursing student a new page to rewrite everything that is on the page that contains the error.

    c. Explain that errors are not acceptable and order the student nurse off the floor.

    d. Explain that the error information is close to being correct and it won't matter because the patient is being discharged anyway.

25. The patient's attorney claims the chart shows that the important procedure was ordered but nothing in the chart shows that it was performed by the nurse. The hospital's attorney places the nurse on the stand to testify that she performed the procedure. What is the judge likely conclude?

    a. The procedure was performed but not charted.

    b. The nurse is lying.

    c. The procedure wasn't performed because it wasn't charted.

    d. Charting the procedure is irrelevant to the case.

26. A common error in recording a patient's intake and output is not including

    a. A heparin flush

    b. Washing hair

c. Discarded medication

    d. Time-release capsule

27. The nurse receives a report from the night shift that the patient's left peripheral IV site is clean and dry. When doing the a.m. assessment, the nurse notes that the IV now appears cool to touch and swollen. The nurse's assessment is best stated as

    a. Left peripheral IV site infiltrated. IV discontinued.

    b. Phlebitis noted to left peripheral IV site.

    c. IV site is clean and dry; no redness or swelling noted.

    d. Infiltrated IV site.

28. You interact with most charting software in the same way as you interact with programs on your home computer.

    a. True

    b. False

29. The date and time entered automatically by the charting software

    a. Is always correct because it is set by the IT department

    b. Must be reviewed and changed by the nurse if it incorrect

    c. Must be reviewed and changed by the IT department if it incorrect

    d. None of the above

30. The patient's nurse using charting software

    a. Can display the patient's previous charts from prior admissions

    b. Must print a copy of each section of the computerized chart after making changes to the chart

    c. Must print a copy of each section of the computerized chart before making changes to the chart

    d. Must provide the nurse manager with a printed copy of the computerized chart at the end of every shift

31. After administering scheduled medication, where would you document it in the chart?

    a. Medication Administration Report

    b. Progress notes

    c. Nurse's notes

    d. Update the care plan

32. Your patient is scheduled to undergo an appendectomy. The physician ordered insertion of a urinary catheter. Before performing the procedure, you inform the patient of the physician's order. The patient refuses permission for you to perform the procedure. What is your best response?

    a. Perform the procedure because the surgical team is in the operating room waiting for the patient.

    b. Don't perform the procedure and then notify the physician that patient refused the procedure.

    c. Explain the necessity of performing the procedure to the patient and then proceed to insert the catheter.

    d. Notify the legal department of the healthcare facility.

33. The nurse is caring for a patient with a nursing diagnosis of impaired skin integrity related to a stage 1 pressure ulcer. The most appropriate goal for this patient is

    a. The patient will not get any more pressure ulcers.

    b. The patient's ulcer will decrease in size from 3 to 2 cm in 1 week.

    c. The patient's ulcer will start to heal.

    d. The patient's skin will not break down.

34. The nurse is caring for a patient with orthostatic hypotension. The nurse's assessment concurs with that diagnosis. The most accurate documentation of that assessment is

    a. Patient appears to be dizzy when standing.

    b. Patient complains of dizziness while ambulating.

    c. Patient's blood pressure lying down is 148/86; when patient stands at bedside, blood pressure is 132/70.

    d. a.m. assessment blood pressure is 150/92.

35. You are automatically logged out of the computer as a security measure.

    a. True

    b. False

36. The nurse is assessing lung sounds. Documentation for the assessment of abnormal breath sounds is best stated as

    a. Lungs clear to ausculation

    b. Upper airway rhonchi heard to anterior chest, clear with coughing, bases clear bilaterally

    c. Rales heard

    d. Rhonchi scattered

37. A student nurse asks how a patient's chart can be used to learn about patient care. The best response is

   a. You can piece together assessments and test results to see how the healthcare provider diagnosed the patient and then see why specific medications and treatments were prescribed to address the patient's problem.

   b. You can look up medical words and tests you see in the chart so you understand what is happening to the patient.

   c. After reviewing the chart, you can call the healthcare provider and ask her why she prescribed medications and treatments that are listed in the chart.

   d. The chart isn't a good tool to use to learn about patient care.

38. Which of the following won't be appropriate to write in a chart?

   a. The patient had a bad day and won't get out of bed to exercise.

   b. The patient in bed, two rails up.

   c. The patient refused to eat breakfast, saying that he wasn't hungry.

   d. 135/70, R 20, P 72, T 98.7.

39. Always circle any medication that wasn't administered and write the reason why it was omitted in the MAR.

   a. True

   b. False

40. The nurse preparing a plan of care for a patient will formulate the plan based on

   a. Medical diagnosis

   b. Nursing diagnosis

   c. Nursing process

   d. Discharge needs

41. What is the major benefit of outsourcing IT tasks?

   a. It is a way to lower IT cost.

   b. It is a way to hire qualified IT technicians.

   c. It is a way to lower IT services.

   d. None of the above.

42. The healthcare facility's computers automatically remove the computerized chart from the screen if there has been no interaction with the chart for a few minutes.

    a. True

    b. False

43. With the To-Do List displayed by charting software you can

    a. Display activity for only your patient

    b. Display activities for your patients that are overdue

    c. Display scheduled activities

    d. All of the above

44. Wifi transmission of patient information can be intercepted.

    a. Yes, but the transmission is limited to the walls of the healthcare facility.

    b. Yes, but patient information is encrypted.

    c. No, because wifi is transmitted using a confidential frequency.

    d. None of the above.

45. The nurse is assessing the patient's wound dressing and sees a large, dark area of red blood on the dressing. The nurse makes a note in the chart describing this as

    a. Purulent drainage

    b. Sanguineous drainage

    c. Scant serosanguineous drainage

    d. Dressing dry and intact

46. What type of care plan uses scientific rationale?

    a. Student and institutional care plans

    b. Institutional care plans

    c. Student care plans

    d. Scientific rationales are never included in a care plan

47. Your patient is an 64-year-old woman admitted 24 hours ago for an exacerbation of her COPD. She is alert, and oriented times 3. Whenever you or the nursing assistant goes into the room she is not very pleasant and yells about the condition of the room and how awful the food is in the hospital. She is a recent widow and lives alone. You met her

daughter briefly when she visited this morning. When you do the morning assessment, on the computer, your comments include

    a. Alert and oriented, recent widow who is being very nasty to the nursing staff.

    b. Alert and oriented times 3. Yelling at nursing staff probably because she is still upset about the recent death of her husband.

    c. Alert and oriented times 3. Recent widow, lives alone; daughter at bedside this morning.

    d. None of the above

48. Medications that are given regularly to the patient to maintain a therapeutic level such as once a day for 7 days are documented as

    a. Double order

    b. PRN

    c. Single order

    d. Schedule medication

49. You enter the room and the patient IV line is disconnected from the patient's arm. The patient tells you, "I don't want this thing hooked up to me anymore." What do you chart?

    a. Entered room at 5:30 p.m. Saline lock not attached to the patient. Pt says, "I don't want this thing hooked up to me anymore."

    b. Entered room. Saline lock not attached to the patient.

    c. Entered room at 5:30 p.m. Saline lock not attached to the patient.

    d. Saline lock not attached to the patient.

50. A student nurse asks how the patient's chart is used for reimbursement of medical expenses. The best response is

    a. The patient's diagnosis is listed in the chart and is compared to Medicare's Diagnosis-Related Group, which is used to determine reimbursements of medical expenses.

    b. The billing department faxes the entire chart to the medical insurance company for review.

    c. The billing department reviews the chart to itemize all the expenses related to caring for the patient.

    d. The chart is not used for reimbursement of medical expenses.

51. At change of shift, the nurse you are relieving forgot to update the patient's chart with the latest vitals. She gives you a slip of paper and asks you to enter it into the chart. What is the best response?

a. Enter the vitals as requested.

b. Say that you'll do it this time only. It is each nurse's responsibility to do his or her own charting

c. Take your own set of vitals and enter it into the chart.

d. Explain that policy requires each nurse to do his or her own charting.

52. The patient is preparing to enter the operating room for routine removal of his gallbladder. He is drowsy from medication that was administered an hour ago. You noticed that the patient did not sign an informed consent for the operation. What is the best response?

a. Proceed with the operation because the physician knows that the patient verbally agreed to the surgery.

b. Have the patient sign the informed consent immediately.

c. Postpone the surgery since the delay will not place the patient at risk.

d. Ask the surgeon or another nurse to witness the patient's response after you ask the patient if he wants to proceed with the surgery.

53. Transferring medical orders to the KARDEX is called taking down orders.

a. True

b. False

54. When is the most appropriate time to create a care plan?

a. When the patient is transferred to the unit

b. At the request of the physician

c. At the request of the nurse supervisor

d. When the patient is admitted

55. The nurse is caring for a postoperative patient with an abdominal incision. At 6 p.m., he gave the patient MS 3 mg IVP for pain described as 9/10 per pain scale and at 6:30 he returned to reevaluate the pain level. The evaluation is best documented by stating:

a. Pain is better.

b. Pain has decreased from the rate 9/10 to rate 4/10.

c. Pain is 4/10

d. Abdominal pain decreased from rate 9/10 to rate 4/10 and described as "bearable"; resting quietly.

56. A patient's chart can be retrieved by patient's medical record number.

a. True

b. False

57. If you discover an error in the Review page
    a. You can return to the chart without saving it and correct the error.
    b. Report the error to the nurse manager, who is authorized to correct the error.
    c. All error corrections must be electronically cosigned by the physician.
    d. None of the above.

58. Weight must be converted to pounds (lbs) in order for the weight to be entered into the chart.
    a. True
    b. False

59. Why is a security filter placed on a computer display?
    a. To filter only patient information from view.
    b. Decrease eye strain.
    c. To prevent viewing from straight in front of the display.
    d. To only allow viewing from straight in front of the display.

60. The nurse is assessing the patient's left lower ankle and notes edema. She presses on the patient's ankle and leaves a deep indentation. She includes in her note the following:
    a. 3+ pitting edema present in left ankle.
    b. Some edema noted.
    c. 1+ edema, no pitting.
    d. Swollen ankle.

61. The healthcare facility determines what items appear on the I&O page of the computerized chart.
    a. True
    b. False

62. If the nurse is unsure of the correct spelling of the patient's name, the nurse
    a. Cannot use charting software to retrieve the patient's chart
    b. Can find the patient's chart by using a partial match search
    c. Must use the patient's ring binder chart
    d. None of the above

63. A member of the healthcare team who is not caring for a patient cannot access the patient's computerized chart.

    a. True

    b. False

64. Most computer charts are divided into sections similar to sections found in a ring binder chart.

    a. True

    b. False

65. Which note below best describes the patient's chest pain?

    a. Patient complains of chest pain and states that it's really bad.

    b. Patient points to chest and says the pain is unbearable.

    c. Complaints of chest pain, 9/10 per pain scale, described by patient as "crushing."

    d. Crushing pain to chest noted.

66. What is the goal of a care plan?

    a. Provide a comprehensive plan for a patient's care.

    b. Provide a check list of tasks for the primary nurse.

    c. Provide a check list of tasks for the nursing staff.

    d. Give the physician guidance for caring for the patient.

67. Always make note of orders that are scheduled to expire at the end of the shift.

    a. True

    b. False

68. The patient arrives in the emergency department with pain in his lower right abdomen. The pain suddenly goes away. He refuses medical care and wants to leave the hospital so he can be at his brother's wedding. The nurse and the physician advise him not to leave because the sudden absence of pain can signify that his condition worsened. He still insists on leaving. What is the best response?

    a. Have the patient sign the Discharge Against Medical Advice form and let him leave.

    b. Have the patient sign the Discharge Against Medical Advice form. Before letting him leave, teach him how to recognize signs that his condition is worsening and where to go for immediate care.

c.   Don't let him go until he is treated.

    d.   Keep explaining to him the risks involved with leaving the hospital.

69. You walk into the room and fined the patient lying on the floor. What do you chart?

    a.   Entered the room at 5:30 p.m. Pt fell out of bed on the floor, left of the bed. Pt was alert, conscious, oriented. Left bed rail down. Right bed rail up.

    b.   Entered the room at 5:30 p.m. Pt on the floor, left of the bed. Pt was alert, conscious, oriented. Left bed rail down. Right bed rail up.

    c.   Entered the room. Pt fell out of bed on the floor left, of the bed. Pt was alert, conscious, oriented. Left bed rail down. Right bed rail up.

    d.   Entered the room. Pt fell out of bed. Pt was alert, conscious, oriented. Left bed rail down. Right bed rail up.

70. A new nurse is having difficulty reading a medical order in the patient's chart. What is the best course of action to take?

    a.   Ask another nurse to help interpret the written order.

    b.   Ask another nurse supervisor to help interpret the written order.

    c.   Call the healthcare provider who wrote the order for clarification.

    d.   Ask the physician on call to interpret the written order.

71. The best way to avoid errors when updating the MAR is to

    a.   Use abbreviates adopted by your healthcare facility

    b.   Update the MAR immediately after you administer medication to a patient

    c.   Dropping the zero following the decimal

    d.   All of the above

72. The macule on the patients left arm is described as a flat, uneven, light brown colored spot.

    a.   True

    b.   False

73. You can request that the healthcare facility insert a new item to the I&O page.

    a.   True

    b.   False

74. The nurse initiates an intervention that

    a.   Has a scientific rationale

    b.   Has a measureable outcome

c. Is specific to the patient

    d. All of the above

75. At the beginning of the shift, balance the opioid inventory control form with a nurse from the outgoing shift

    a. True

    b. False

76. The purpose of giving a report to the new primary nurse is to

    a. Provide a complete and thorough history of the patient

    b. Quickly bring the nurse up-to-date on the patient's status

    c. Give a detailed status of all the patient's medical tests

    d. Introduce the nurse to the patient's preferences

77. The nurse can display a list of the nurse's patients by diagnoses.

    a. True

    b. False

78. The nurse is evaluating the plan of care for a patient and determines that a problem still exists. The FIRST revision to the plan of care is

    a. The problem

    b. The intervention

    c. The nursing diagnosis

    d. The goal

79. A new nurse asks what abbreviates can be used in a chart. The best response is?

    a. Review hospital policy.

    b. Only use abbreviations that are found in standard nursing textbooks.

    c. Never use any abbreviations.

    d. Always use abbreviations to save time and space in the chart.

80. A 45-year-old man is being treated for gout. He is sleeping when his 21-year-old son arrives to visit. The son is concerned about his father's condition and demands to see his father's chart. The best response is?

    a. Explain that you are not permitted to do so because of patient confidentiality laws and reassure him that his father is receiving proper care.

    b. Show him the chart under your supervision.

c. Show him the chart.

    d. Call security.

81. A physician writes a DNR order for your patient who is terminally ill with cancer. Forty-eight hours later the patient shows signs of severe respiratory distress. She is conscious and oriented. She indicates that she wants to be placed on a respirator. What is the best response?

    a. Call the physician and prepare for her to be placed on the respirator.

    b. Tell her that her physician has written a DNR order.

    c. Notify the legal department of the healthcare facility.

    d. Begin CPR.

82. The physician has written a DNR order for your terminally ill cancer patient. The patient's family are the only ones in the room when the patient becomes unconscious. Family members tell you that right before he fell unconscious, the patient said that he wanted everything done so he could live. What is the best response?

    a. Tell the family that the physician wrote a DNR order.

    b. Call the legal department of your facility.

    c. Remove the DNR order from the chart.

    b. Call another nurse into the room to witness the family's statement.

83. The features of charting software that you can access depend on the right assigned to your ID.

    a. True

    b. False

84. Entry in a computerized chart

    a. Cannot be cosigned

    b. Is not accepted as the official medical record for a patient

    c. Is a tool used to print a patient's chart

    d. None of the above

85. Anyone with access to the healthcare facility's computers can access a patient's computerized chart.

    a. True

    b. False

86. Which of the following cannot access a patient's medical records?

    a. The patient's primary nurse

    b. The LPN assigned to the patient

c.   The healthcare facility's IT department

    d.   The nurse manager of the patient's unit

87. The patient's family has a right to see the patient's chart.

    a.   True

    b.   False

88. A mistake in the MAR can be erased and corrected by the nurse who made the error.

    a.   True

    b.   False

89. Charting software provides a list of assessments that the nurse is expected to perform on a patient.

    a.   True

    b.   False

90. When your patient requests to view his chart

    a.   Consult the healthcare facility's policy for providing patients with their charts.

    b.   Make a copy and give the patient his chart.

    c.   Hand the patient his ring binder chart and wait until the patient finishes reviewing it.

    d.   Hand the patient his ring binder chart and return later to pickup the chart.

91. When a healthcare facility converts to computerized charting

    a.   All charts can be displayed using charting software.

    b.   Only new charts and previous charts that have been converted to electronic format can be displayed using charting software.

    c.   New charts and all previous charts can be displayed using charting software.

    d.   None of the above.

92. Computerized charts are more reliable than ring binder charts.

    a.   True

    b.   False

93. Members of the healthcare team are no longer responsible for the accuracy of computerized charts because they don't write their signature on the chart.

    a.   True

    b.   False

94. What reasons have healthcare facilities given for not adopting computerized charting?

     a. Expense

     b. Lack of universally accepted charting software

     c. Acceptance by the healthcare team

     d. All of the above

95. Computerized medical records are secured by data encryption.

     a. True

     b. False

96. A risk of viewing a computerized chart on the screen is

     a. The computer might automatically log you off.

     b. Anyone behind the screen can read the patient's medical record.

     c. You are unable to take a copy of the chart to the bedside.

     d. None of the above.

97. You are assigned rights to features of charting software based on your need to care for your patient.

     a. True

     b. False

98. If the computer automatically logs you out

     a. Log back in.

     b. Call the IT department for assistance.

     c. Use your nurse manager's ID.

     d. Use your nursing assistant's ID.

99. You can print a portion of your patient's chart using charting software.

     a. True

     b. False

100. You can use charting software to look up a patient by

     a. Medical record number

     b. Account number

     c. Name

     d. All of the above

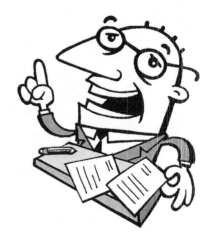

Answers to Quizzes

Chapter 1

1. d. Explain that policy requires each nurse to do their own charting.

2. a. Explain that errors occur and then draw a single line through the error and initial it.

3. d. An incident report.

4. c. The treatment wasn't performed because it wasn't charted.

5. a. Review hospital policy.

6. c. Call the healthcare provider who wrote the order for clarification.

7. a. Medication Administration Report.

8. a. The patient had a bad day and won't get out of bed to exercise.

9. a. The patient's diagnosis is listed in the chart and is compared to Medicare's Diagnosis-Related Group, which is used to determine reimbursements of medical expenses.

10. a. You can piece together assessments and test results to see how the healthcare provider diagnosed the patient and then see why specific medications and treatments were prescribed to address the patient's problem.

Chapter 2

1. b. Entered the room at 5:30 p.m. Pt on the floor, left of the bed. Pt was alert, conscious, oriented. Left bed rail down. Right bed rail up.

2. a. Entered room at 5:30 p.m. Saline lock not attached to the patient. Pt says, "I don't want this thing hooked up to me anymore."

3. c. Determine if the physician has written a DNR order.

4. b. Don't perform the procedure and then notify the physician that patient refused the procedure.

5. a. Call the physician and prepare for her to be placed on the respirator.

6. c. Postpone the surgery since the delay will not place the patient at risk.

7. b. Write an incident report.

8. b. Have the patient sign the discharge Against Medical Advice form. Before letting him leave, teach him how to recognize signs that his condition is worsening and where to go for immediate care.

9. b. Call the legal department of your facility.

10. a. Explain that you are not permitted to do so because of patient confidentiality laws and reassure him that his father is receiving proper care.

Chapter 3

1. b. Intake and Output form

2. b. Quickly bring the nurse up-to-date on the patient's status.

3. a. A heparin flush

4. b. False

5. a. True

6. d. All of the above

7. a. True

8. d. Schedule Medication

9. a. True

10. a. True

Chapter 4

1. b. The intervention

2. c. Nursing process

3. d. All of the above

4. b. The patient's ulcer will decrease in size from 3 to 2 cm in 1 week

5. a. Assessment

6. d. When the patient is admitted

7. c. Following assessment of the patient

8. b. The primary nurse

9. a. Provide a comprehensive plan for a patient's care

10. c. Student care plans

Chapter 5

1. c. Alert, disoriented to place, responses inappropriate, demonstrates facial grimacing with incisional palpation, pain level indeterminable

2. b. Sanguineous drainage

3. a. 3+ pitting edema present to left ankle

4. a. True

5. c. Patient's blood pressure lying down is 148/86; when patient stands at bedside blood pressure is 132/70.

6. b. Upper airway rhonchi heard to anterior chest, clear with coughing, bases clear bilaterally

7. a. Left peripheral IV site swollen and cool to the touch. IV discontinued.

8. c. Complains of chest pain, 9/10 per pain scale, described by patient as "crushing."

9. d. Abdominal pain decreased from rate 9/10 to rate 4/10 and described as "bearable"; resting quietly.

10. c. Sleepy but arousable.

Chapter 6

1. a. It is a way to lower IT cost.
2. d. Only to allow viewing from straight in front of the display
3. c. As your hometown
4. a. True
5. a. True
6. a. Converting information into meaningless information using a key and mathematical formula
7. a. True
8. b. Yes, but patient information is encrypted.
9. a. True
10. a. True

Chapter 7

1. d. All of the above
2. a. True
3. a. Can display the patient's previous charts from prior admissions
4. a. True
5. a. True
6. b. Can find the patient's chart by using a partial match search
7. a. True
8. c. Is stored in a central database
9. a. True
10. a. True

Chapter 8

1. b. Must be reviewed and changed by the nurse if it is incorrect
2. b. False
3. b. Is based on the date and time scheduled by the order

4. a. True

5. b. False

6. a. You can return to the chart without saving it and correct the error.

7. a. True

8. d. All of the above.

9. a. True

10. a. True

Chapter 9

1. c. The order in which the assessment is listed in charting software

2. a. Add a comment to the assessment

3. c. Click the word or check box to unselect it

4. a. True

5. a. True

6. d. All of the above

7. b. False

8. b. The healthcare team can review the chart anywhere within the healthcare facility's computer network.

9. a. True

10. a. True

Chapter 10

1. a. Is a series of dark bars of various thicknesses that represents a unique number.

2. b. Notify the physician personally, enter a comment in the charting software, and set the exclamation flag.

3. a. Any member of the healthcare team can access the medication record from within the healthcare facility's computer network.

4. a. True

5. b. False

6. c. Overwrite the values displayed by the charting software.

7. a. True

8. b. Call the pharmacy and ask that they deliver the medication

9. a. True

10. b. False

Chapter 11

1. b. A symptom

2. c. An order that specifies a pattern of facts that if exists authorizes the nurse to write a specific order for the patient without obtaining permission from the patient's primary physician.

3. c. A member of the healthcare team who is authorized to write an order.

4 a. True

5. a. True

6. d. All of the above

7. a. True

8. a. Verbal

9. b. False

10. a. True

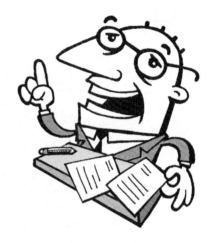

Answers to
Final Exam

1. b. Write an incident report.

2. a. Assessment

3. False

4. b. Is based on the date and time scheduled by the order

5. d. None of the above

6. c. As your hometown

7. c. Alert, disoriented to place, responses inappropriate, demonstrates facial grimacing with incisional palpation, pain level indeterminable

8. d. All of the above

9. c. Determine if the physician has written a DNR order

10. a. True

11. d. An incident report

12. b. Intake and Output form

13. b. False

14. d. All of the above

15. b. False

16. a. Converting information into meaningless information using a key and mathematical formula

17. c. Patient's blood pressure lying down is 148/86; when patient stands at bedside, blood pressure is 132/70.

18. c. Following assessment of the patient

19. a. True

20. b. False

21. b. False

22. c. Sleepy but arousable

23. b. The nursing assistant

24. a. Explain that errors occur and then draw a single line through the error and initial it.

25. c. The procedure wasn't performed because it wasn't charted.

26. a. A heparin flush

27. a. Left peripheral IV site infiltrated. IV discontinued.

28. a. True

29. b. Must be reviewed and changed by the nurse if it incorrect

30. a. Can display the patient's previous charts from prior admissions

31. a. Medication Administration Report

32. b. Don't perform the procedure and then notify the physician that that patient refused the procedure.

33. b. The patient's ulcer will decrease in size from 3 to 2 cm in 1 week

34. c. Patient's blood pressure lying down is 148/86; when patient stands at bedside, blood pressure is 132/70.

35. a. True

36. b. Upper airway rhonchi heard to anterior chest, clear with coughing, bases clear bilaterally

37. a. You can piece together assessments and test results to see how the healthcare provider diagnosed the patient and then see why specific

medications and treatments were prescribed to address the patient's problem.

38. a. The patient had a bad day and won't get out of bed to exercise.

39. a. True

40. c. Nursing process

41. a. It is a way to lower IT cost.

42. a. True

43. d. All of the above

44. b. Yes, but patient information is encrypted

45. b. Sanguineous drainage

46. c. Student care plans

47. c. Alert, and oriented times 3. Recent widow, lives alone; daughter at bedside this morning

48. d. Schedule medication

49. a. Entered room at 5:30 p.m. Saline lock not attached to the patient. Pt says, "I don't want this thing hooked up to me anymore."

50. a. The patient's diagnosis is listed in the chart and is compared to Medicare's Diagnosis-Related Group, which is used to determine reimbursements of medical expenses.

51. d. Explain that policy requires each nurse to do his or her own charting.

52. c. Postpone the surgery since the delay will not place the patient at risk.

53. a. True

54. d. When the patient is admitted

55. d. Abdominal pain decreased from rate 9/10 to rate 4/10 and described as "bearable"; resting quietly.

56. a. True

57. a. You can return to the chart without saving it and correct the error.

58. b. False

59. d. To only allow viewing from straight in front of the display

60. a. 3+ pitting edema present in left ankle

61. a. True

62. b. Can find the patient's chart by using a partial match search

63. a. True

64. a. True

65. c. Complaints of chest pain, 9/10 per pain scale, described by patient as "crushing"

66. a. Provide a comprehensive plan for a patient's care

67. a. True

68. b. Have the patient sign the Discharge Against Medical Advice form. Before letting him leave, teach him how to recognize signs that his condition is worsening and where to go for immediate care.

69. b. Entered the room at 5:30 p.m. Pt on the floor left of the bed. Pt was alert, conscious, oriented. Left bed rail down. Right bed rail up.

70. c. Call the healthcare provider who wrote the order for clarification.

71. d. All of the above

72. a. True

73. a. True

74. d. All of the above

75. a. True

76. b. Quickly bring the nurse up-to-date on the patient's status

77. a. True

78. b. The intervention

79. a. Review hospital policy

80. a. Explain that you are not permitted to do so because of patient confidentiality laws and reassure him that his father is receiving proper care.

81. a. Call the physician and prepare for her to be placed on the respirator.

82. b. Call the legal department of your facility.

83. a. True

84. d. None of the above.

85. b. False

86. c. The healthcare facility's IT department

87. b. False

88. b. False

89. a. True

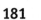

90. a. Consult the healthcare facility's policy for providing patients with their charts

91. b. Only new charts and previous charts that have been converted to electronic format can be displayed using charting software.

92. b. False

93. b. False

94. d. All of the above

95. a. True

96. b. Anyone behind the screen can read the patient's medical record.

97. a. True

98. a. Log back in

99. a. True

100. d. All of the above

INDEX

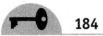

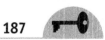

CPSIA information can be obtained
at www.ICGtesting.com
Printed in the USA
BVOW10s1231280217
477365BV00005B/21/P